Smoothies for Life

Smoothies for Life

Yummy, Fun, and Nutritious

Daniella Chace
Maureen Keane

 THREE RIVERS PRESS • NEW YORK

Published by Three Rivers Press, New York, New York.
Member of the Crown Publishing Group, a division of Random House, Inc.
www.crownpublishing.com

THREE RIVERS PRESS and the Tugboat design are registered trademarks of Random House, Inc.

Originally published by Prima Publishing, Roseville, California, in 1998.

A per serving nutritional breakdown is provided for each recipe. Each recipe is treated as one serving. If a range is given for an ingredient amount, the breakdown is based on the smaller number. If a choice of ingredients is given in an ingredient listing, the breakdown is calculated using the first choice. Nutritional content may vary depending on the specific brands or types of ingredients used. "Optional" ingredients or those for which no specific amount is stated are not included in the breakdown.

This book is not meant to be a substitute for medical counseling or a guide for those on restricted diets. Readers with restricted diets should follow the guidance of their physician. The author and Random House, Inc., shall have neither liability nor responsibility to any person or entity with respect to any loss, damage, or injury caused or alleged to be caused directly or indirectly by the information contained in this book.

Printed in the United States of America

Library of Congress Cataloging-in-Publication Data

Chace, Daniella.
    Smoothies for life : yummy, fun, nutritious / Daniella Chace and Maureen Keane.
        p.   cm.
    Includes index.
    1. Fruit drinks.   2. Smoothies (Beverages).   I. Keane, Maureen.
II. Title
TX815.C45 1998
641.8'75—dc21   98-2552
                                                                          CIP

ISBN 0-7615-1340-X
    15

First Edition

Contents

Making Smoothies

Smoothies are thick drinks made in the blender or food processor from whole or frozen foods and liquids such as milk or juice. They are unusually popular at the moment, because they are delicious and can be consumed on-the-go. Breakfast smoothies can be drunk on the drive to work. Lunch smoothies can be drunk at the desk easily. On the weekend, they offer a quick meal replacement as you run to children's soccer games, for example. They are versatile, they do not require the purchase of expensive equipment, and they are quick and easy to make.

SMOOTHIE EQUIPMENT

You probably have all the equipment you need now to make great smoothies: a blender or a food processor. If you have both, you may want to experiment to see which gives you the best results. If you are going to buy a new blender, invest in the most powerful motor you can find. The size of the motor will determine how well and how long the appliance will work. Look for a strong, easy-to-clean base. Do you really need all those speed buttons? Prying dried fruit out of all those sharp corners quickly gets tedious. Maureen's favorite blender has only two speeds, and she has never really needed more than that.

Some blenders come with glass containers, which are easier to clean and look better longer. Plastic is much lighter in weight for those with strength problems, but they are more easily scratched and stained. Which one you buy is of a personal preference.

HOW TO MAKE SMOOTHIES

It is very hard to go wrong when making a smoothie. Usually, you can let your taste buds make the choice of ingredients. We will offer a few suggestions to get you started. Drink smoothies within ten minutes of making them because the water-soluble nutrients will begin to oxidize and the enzymes of fresh fruit will begin to brown the produce after about ten minutes. Also, the ingredients may begin to separate, making the smoothie less than appealing.

Smoothies made during the winter will require less frozen components for thickness than will smoothies made in the heat of summer. Simply add a little water, juice, or milk to smoothies that are too thick. Add ice cubes or frozen fruit to smoothies that are too thin.

SMOOTHIES FOR CHILDREN

Smoothies are a great way to get your child to eat healthy foods. For example, healthy soy foods that your child would never eat on their own become favorite foods when mixed into a smoothie. Just a word of caution: *Never* add herbs or food supplements to smoothies for children without checking with your pediatrician for dosages. What can be life saving for an adult can be life threatening to a child.

Children under the age of two years should never eat honey even if it is pasteurized. Honey can transmit heat-resistant botulism spores that can be very dangerous to children. Honey also can adversely affect blood sugar levels. Protein powders are not substitutes for baby formula and should never be given to infants.

THE NEVER-ENDING SMOOTHIE

This chapter will help you design your own smoothie recipes based on your individual tastes, needs, and wants. To make the perfect smoothie, start with a 1/2 cup to 1 cup of a liquid base. Add 1 cup of fruit, flavoring to taste, supplements as needed, and then blend until smooth. Pour the finished smoothie into a tall glass and then sit back and enjoy. That's all there is to it! Don't be afraid to experiment. Almost any soft fruit or vegetable juice tastes great when added to a smoothie. Each recipe makes a single serving from 8 to 16 ounces.

LIQUID BASE

Use 1/2 to 1 cup

The milk of your choice adds a creamy note, yogurt adds a tang, and tofu adds thickness. Coconut milk adds a tropical flavor to any smoothie, but it is very high in fat. Regular coconut milk contains about ten grams of fat per each two-tablespoon serving! Much of that fat is saturated. Lowfat coconut milk is now available in most grocery stores and specialty markets. It contains about two grams of fat per each two-tablespoon serving.

Whole dairy milk is rich in saturated fat, the kind of fat that will promote heart disease, therefore you should use only 1 percent or fat-free milk and yogurt. Soy milk, on the other hand, is made with polyunsaturated fats that prevent heart disease, so whole soy milk and yogurt are preferable.

Goat's milk is available in the dairy case of many grocery stores and health food stores. As an alternative to cow's milk, it may be helpful to those with dairy allergies, however, it does contain lactose, the milk sugar many people cannot digest, and milk fat, which is associated with heart disease.

Nut and seed milk can be used as the liquid portion of the recipe. You can buy nut and seed milks at health food stores or make your own. You'll find a recipe at the end of this chapter, where you'll also find recipes for oat milk and rice milk.

Vegetables and fruit juice add flavor and nutrients to the base of a drink. Tomato juice or puree, for example, makes a good start for a

Coconut milk
Cow's milk (1 percent, skim, non-fat, buttermilk, acidophilus added, and others)
Cow's milk yogurt (nonfat plain or flavored)
Cranberry juice cocktail
Frozen yogurt (lowfat and nonfat)
Fruit juice (grapefruit, orange, apple, prune, and others)
Ice cream (lowfat and nonfat)
Ice cubes
Ice milk
Mint tea and other herbal teas
Nut and seed milk (almond, sesame seed, and others)
Oat milk
Rice milk
Sherbet
Sorbet
Soy milk (whole or lowfat, plain or flavored)
Soy yogurt (whole or lowfat, plain or flavored)
Sparkling water
Tea (green or black)
Tofu (soft or silken)
Vegetable juice (tomato, carrot, and others)
Water, filtered

homemade V8-type drink. The best flavor comes from freshly made vegetable juices (dust off that juicer!), but canned or locally bottled vegetable juices can be substituted.

If you want a smoothie that is lower in calories, use filtered water, tea, or ice as the base. Filtered water should be used for making ice cubes, mixing with juices, and as a base for drinks. Use a solid carbon filter for municipal (city) waters. Solid carbon filters reduce chlorine, heavy metals, and asbestos particles. Use a distiller for well water to be sure all the living organisms are removed.

When brewing fresh tea, steep the leaves in boiled water for a few minutes (remember that the longer the tea brews, the higher its caffeine content). Strain out the leaves, cool, and use the tea in your smoothie.

FRUITS

Use 1 cup

The easiest way to make smoothies is to use frozen fruit that is stored in the freezer. It's always handy and never spoils. The more frozen fruit

Apples, cored and peeled
Applesauce
Apricots, pitted and peeled
Avocados, pitted and peeled
Bananas, peeled
Blackberries
Blueberries
Cherries, pitted
Cranberries
Currants
Dates, pitted and soaked
Figs, fresh chopped
Gooseberries
Grapefruits, peeled and seeded
Grapes, seedless varieties
Kiwis, peeled
Lemons, peeled and seeded
Limes, peeled
Loganberries

Mangoes, peeled and seeded
Marionberries
Melons (such as cantaloupes,
   watermelon), rind and seeds
   removed
Nectarines, pitted and peeled
Oranges, peeled and seeded
Papayas, pitted and peeled
Passion fruit, peeled
Peaches, pitted and peeled
Pears, cored and peeled
Pineapples, peeled
Plums, pitted and peeled
Pomegranates, seeds only
Prunes, pitted and soaked
Raisins, soaked
Raspberries
Strawberries
Tangerines, peeled and seeded

that is used, the thicker the smoothie. Very thick smoothies can be served with a spoon as a soft dessert. During the winter, when icy, thick smoothies are too cold to be appealing, we use room-temperature canned peaches, apricots, papaya, mango, and applesauce to add thickness. Dried fruits can be used as well. Soak dried fruit, such as raisins, dates, and apricot slices, in fruit juice or water overnight, and then puree until smooth. They add trace minerals and flavor as well as fiber.

Bananas are one of the most popular smoothies ingredients. When a banana is frozen, ice crystals form, which change the viscous texture to a creamy one. A blended frozen banana has the smooth rich texture of ice cream, and one frozen banana is a nutritious substitute for a scoop of ice cream or frozen yogurt in a smoothie. Peel a few ripe bananas, cut them into two-inch pieces, and put them in a plastic bag. Store them in the freezer so they are readily available. We like to use one-half banana for every one cup of fruit. If a smoothie comes out too thick, add more liquid and blend again.

FLAVORS

Use the recommended amounts, or to taste

Spices add not only flavor but also nutritional value. Many are sources of potent antioxidants. Frozen juice concentrate adds flavor and sweetness to smoothies thickened with silken tofu or yogurt.

Natural sweeteners can be used to give smoothies extra flavor or to help cover up the taste of added supplements. Dates, fruit sweeteners, fruit juice concentrate, molasses, maple syrup, honey, and Sucanat will add sweetness. Guava nectar, mango nectar, mint syrup, strawberry juice, or flavored syrups can be used in small quantities to add tremendous flavor. Yogurt is generally used to add protein, calcium, and beneficial microflora to smoothies. Add a tablespoon of sweetener, such as honey, to take the tart edge off a yogurt-based smoothie. When adding sweeteners, remember that they also add calories and simple sugars and should be used sparingly by those with diabetes, hypoglycemia, or syndrome X.

Almond extract
Apple pie spice
Cardamom, ground
Carob
Cinnamon, ground
Cloves, ground
Cocoa powder
Coconut, grated or shredded
Coconut extract
Coffee (instant powder)
Flavored syrups
Frozen fruit juice concentrate
Fruit juice concentrate (1 to
    3 tablespoons)
Fruit sweeteners
Ginger, fresh (2-inch piece, peeled
    and crushed) or ground

Guava nectar
Honey
Lemon (1/2 lemon, peeled
    and seeded)
Licorice
Lime (1/2 lime, peeled)
Mango nectar
Maple syrup
Mint syrup
Molasses
Nutmeg, ground
Pumpkin pie spice
Strawberry juice
Sucanat
Vanilla extract

OTHER INGREDIENTS

Cereals and Grains

You don't have to limit yourself, however, to fruits and juices. Cold cereals, such as Grapenuts, shredded wheat, granola, and brown rice cereals, can be added to a smoothie. Just put cold cereals in the blender cup with a liquid base and soak for one minute before mixing. Cooked grains, such as oats, brown rice, kasha, or kamut, can also be added to the blender. Cereals add fiber, complex carbohydrates, and texture.

Brown rice (cooked)
Brown rice cereal
Granola
Grapenuts

Kamut (cooked)
Kasha (cooked)
Oats (cooked)
Shredded wheat

Nuts and Seeds

These ingredients add texture, heart-healthy monounsaturated fats, and fat-soluble vitamins. There are several way to add nuts and seeds to your smoothie. Finely ground nuts can be added to thick smoothies. Nut milk can provide the liquid base. See the recipe at the end of the chapter. Nut or seed butters blend easily into any mixture.

Almonds
Brazil nuts
Hazelnuts (also called filberts)
Nut butters (almond, peanut,
    cashew, and others)
Peanuts
Pecans

Pine nuts
Pumpkin seeds
Sesame seeds
Sunflower seeds
Tahini (ground sesame seeds)
Walnuts

CULINARY AND MEDICINAL HERBS

The culinary herbs (herbs used in cooking to impart flavor) used in this book are garlic, onion, ginger root, peppermint, and peppers. They can be used raw. Black and green tea is actually an herbal infusion since the herb (the tea leaf) is soaked in boiled water and discarded. Although these herbs have many medicinal qualities they can be consumed in greater amounts than medicinal herbs.

The rest of the herbs mentioned here are medicinal herbs. We do not recommend using fresh or died herbs in these recipes. Not only are many herbs not palatable but you have no way of knowing how much of the active ingredient is present. In health food stores, medicinal herbs are available as tinctures or extracts.

Tinctures are made by soaking the herb in a mixture of alcohol and water. These solvents are then separated from the herb yielding the tincture. Tinctures can also be made by diluting fluid extracts with alcohol. Tinctures are sold in glass bottles with droppers. The directions on the label will tell you how many drops to add to your smoothie.

Extracts are much more concentrated than tinctures. They are also made by soaking herbs in solvents. After the tincture is pressed out of the herb, all of the solvent is then removed from the tincture. This leaves only the material extracted from the herb. Liquid extracts are made by dissolving this extract in water and alcohol. Solid extracts are made by grinding the extract into powder.

Many herbal extracts have a bitter flavor. Licorice, an herb with a sweet taste, is often added to liquid extracts to mask their bitter taste. Look for herbal extracts sold in convenient serving-sized packets. The extract is premeasured and sealed until you open it.

Astragalus	Kava
Echinacea	Licorice
Ginger	Peppermint
Ginkgo biloba	Silymarin (milk thistle)
Ginseng	Tea
Goldenseal	

Solid extracts can be purchased in a variety of forms. Buy those that are available as powders. These extracts are designed to be more palatable than extracts packaged in capsules.

Always buy only standardized extracts. This is your assurance that you are getting a potent product.

SUPPLEMENTS

Thick smoothies offer the opportunity to add a variety of food supplements. The amounts listed here are only rough estimates, since the recommended dosage varies widely according to the concentration of the product. Always read the label to be sure of what you are adding.

Some of these supplements are an acquired taste. We recommend that you start with a small amount and gradually increase each day until you are at the recommended level. The gritty texture of many soy supplements can be reduced by mixing them with a thick fruit, such as a banana or canned peaches. The bitter taste of many herbs can be masked with flavoring agents.

Just because you are drinking your herbs as part of a sweet shake does not mean that these potent chemicals should not be respected. Add only herbs with which you are familiar. If you take any prescription drug, check with your physician or pharmacist about possible interactions. Some herbs should not be taken on a regular basis. Some should not be taken by people with heart disease, hypertension, or edema. More is never better. Never exceed the recommended dose without your physician's recommendation.

Do you often add supplements to your smoothies? Mix them ahead of time and store the mixture in small airtight containers or bags until needed. This can be a real time-saver when making a quick lunch smoothie or breakfast smoothie. Here's one example of a premixed powered supplement:

1 scoop protein powder
1 tablespoon brewer's yeast
1 tablespoon flaxseed powder
1 teaspoon vitamin C powder
1 teaspoon acidophilus

Acidophilus (1 teaspoon)
Algae (1 teaspoon)
Amino acid powders (varies)
Bee pollen (1 tablespoon)
Brewer's yeast (1 tablespoon)
Calcium liquid (1 tablespoon)
Chlorella (1 teaspoon)
Chlorophyll liquid or powder
    (1 tablespoon)
Creatine (1/2 teaspoon)
Dulse (1/2 teaspoon)
Flaxseed oil (1 teaspoon)
Flaxseed powder (1 tablespoon)
Kelp powder (1/2 teaspoon)
Lecithin granules (1 tablespoon)

Magnesium liquid or powder
    (varies)
Medium chain triglyceride
    (MCT) oil
Oat bran (1 tablespoon)
Propolis (1 tablespoon)
Protein powder (3 tablespoons),
    plain or flavored
Psyllium seed powder (1 teaspoon)
Rice bran/polish (1 teaspoon)
Spirulina (1 teaspoon)
Vitamin C powder (1 teaspoon)
Wheat bran (1 teaspoon)
Wheat germ (1 tablespoon)

HEALTHFUL SMOOTHIE INGREDIENTS

Your smoothie is only as healthful as the ingredients you put into it. Ice cream and whole milk may taste great, but they also add harmful amounts of saturated fat. Sherbet and other frozen confections contribute flavor but also add large amounts of empty sugar. Make your smoothies as inviting to the inside of your body as they are to your outer taste buds, by using pure, whole ingredients whenever possible. Fresh whole fruits add fiber, vitamins, minerals, flavonoids, carotenoids, and other bioactive compounds. These substances work together to prevent cancer, heart disease, stroke, osteoporosis, and diabetes and help to treat irregularity, menopausal symptoms, and bacterial and viral infections. They can aid you in buffing up or slimming down.

Any soft fruit that can be blended can be added to smoothies. You are not limited to the ingredients mentioned here. Don't forget that some vegetable juice can also be added to smoothies. Vegetable juice makes a healthful natural "supplement," so do not hesitate to add green juices to your smoothies. The idea that vegetable and fruit juices do not mix is an old wives' tale. Your body will welcome their nutrition.

In the past, nutritionists have focused on the vitamins and minerals found in fruit, but recently the attention has shifted to their phytochemical content. Phytochemicals are compounds that have a medicinal effect in the body. Much of the preventative properties of fruits and vegetables against heart disease and cancer come from these agents rather than from the vitamins and minerals they contain. So don't hesitate to use fruits that are not considered to be nutrient-dense. They also have unique benefits to offer.

FRUIT AND VEGETABLE INGREDIENTS

Apples

As juice, frozen juice concentrate, applesauce, dried slices, and fresh (peeled and cored)
Apples are a source of pectin and potassium.

Rich in the soluble fiber pectin, apples contribute to blood sugar and cholesterol regulation and promote the growth and maintenance of beneficial intestinal flora necessary for a healthy colon. Pectin also aids in the reduction of blood cholesterol and may help to prevent certain cancers in the colon. Apples are also a good source of the following: polyphenols, substances that have antiviral and antibacterial properties; glutathione, a potent antioxidant that helps prevent heart disease and cancer; and malic acid, a fruit acid that is a powerful chelator or binder of heavy metals, such as cadmium and lead. Apples are useful in normalizing colon function. The pectin acts as a binder, decreasing the severity of diarrhea, while its sorbitol content acts as a natural laxative.

In smoothies, apple juice lends sweetness without an overpowering flavor. Frozen apples and applesauce make smoothies thicker, and dried apples add body to thin mixtures. Always peel and core fresh apples before adding them to your smoothie.

Apricots

As juice, dried slices, peeled and pitted, fresh or frozen, without sugar, and canned
Apricots are a source of provitamin A, fiber, and potassium.

Apricots are wonderful sources of beta carotene. This pigment is changed into vitamin A by the body. Preformed vitamin A can be toxic in large amounts, but beta carotene is only transformed into vitamin A when the body needs the nutrient. This makes beta carotene a nontoxic source of this important fat-soluble vitamin. Vitamin A is necessary for vision, growth, reproduction, the differentiation of cells, and the soundness of the immune system. Aside from its vitamin A activity, beta carotene is famous in its own right as an antioxidant. Antioxidants protect your genetic material and cell membranes from the free radical–induced damage that initiates heart disease and cancers. Apricots are also a good source of potassium, a trace mineral that research has shown to lower blood pressure. Dried apricots are the most concentrated source of beta carotene and also supply iron and copper.

To add dried apricots to a smoothie, first soak the slices in water for a few minutes, or if they are very dry, soak them overnight, then process until they are a smooth puree. Add the remaining smoothie ingredients to your blender and continue with the recipe. Apricot puree adds body to thin drinks. Canned apricots add thickness and smoothness to drinks and are a good alternative to frozen fruit in the winter.

Avocados

Fresh (pitted and peeled)
Avocados are a source of potassium, folic acid, vitamin E, oleic acid, and protein.

Avocados are often thought of as a vegetable but are really a fruit. They are rich in oleic acid, containing a higher percentage of this healthy monounsaturated fatty acid than even olive oil. Oleic acid is the fatty acid credited with the decrease in heart disease and cancer seen with the Mediterranean diet. This fat makes avocados a concentrated source of calories for those who need to increase their caloric intake without adding dangerous saturated fats.

Avocados are one of the richest studied sources of glutathione, a part of the glutathione peroxidase enzyme. This enzyme is used by cells of the heart, liver, lungs, and blood to defend themselves from the damage of free radicals. The vitamin E found in avocados enhances the anticancer effects of glutathione.

Half an avocado contains a whopping 600 mg of the electrolyte potassium, which is more of this mineral than is found in a whole banana. A high intake of potassium is associated with a decreased risk of developing high blood pressure.

The ripe flesh of an avocado has the consistency of firm butter and a taste reminiscent of nuts. Peel and pit avocados before placing them in the blender. They add a wickedly rich texture to drinks.

Bananas

Peeled fresh or frozen
Bananas are a source of pyridoxine (B6), potassium,
    magnesium, folate, and pectin.

This tropical fruit is a good source of pectin, a soluble fiber that decreases the risk of heart disease and some colon cancers. Bananas protect the stomach from excess acid and aid in the healing of peptic ulcers.

A study in Cleveland found that vitamin B6 deficiency may increase the risk of heart disease. The researchers looked at vitamin B6 levels in 304 male and female patients with heart disease and 231 healthy controls. They found that levels of vitamin B6 below 20 nmol/L increased the risk of coronary heart disease more than fourfold.

Bananas are a good source of potassium, an electrolyte that is often lost during exercise or with the use of diuretics. High potassium intake is linked to a lower risk of developing hypertension.

Add a few pieces of a frozen banana to smoothies for a creamy, milk shake-textured drink. Fresh bananas add thickness and body to smoothies.

Blackberries

Fresh or frozen without added sugar
Blackberries are a source of potassium, manganese,
    and insoluble fiber.

The blackberry is an aggregate fruit made up of small, purplish-black drupes. Like all berries, it is rich in the antioxidant flavonoids. Finnish researchers found in a study of 5,133 men and women that those whose diets were highest in flavonoids were less likely to die from coronary disease than those whose diets contained less of the antioxidant substances. The benefit was most pronounced in women. Women who consumed the most flavonoids were about half as likely to die of heart disease as those who consumed the lowest amount. In men, those who consumed the most flavonoids were about 25 percent less likely to die of heart disease than those who ate the least.

Blackberries also are rich in potassium, the trace mineral that reduces high blood pressure, and in saponins, which are compounds that can reduce cholesterol levels. Blackberries and blueberries are also a very good source of natural aspirin (salicylates) and in the test tube kill viruses.

Fresh or frozen blackberries can be added to smoothies. A few frozen berries add a deep purple color to smoothies.

Blueberries

Fresh or frozen without sugar and dried
Blueberries are a source of vitamin C, potassium, magnesium, and the reddish-blue pigment anthocyanins.

Blueberries belong to the same genus as cranberries and contain the same unknown "cranberry chemical" that prevents the adhesion of bacteria to the wall of the bladder. Thus they have the same ability to prevent bladder infections. Blueberries are one of the highest sources of salicylate, a natural aspirin-like compound that has been shown to reduce inflammation and prevent blood coagulation. These properties make this fruit a good choice for those with heart disease and diseases that cause inflammation.

In the test tube, blueberries have shown antiviral activity. Dried blueberries are a traditional treatment for diarrhea.

Fresh, frozen, or dried blueberries can be added whole to smoothies, where they impart a mild sweetness and a deep blue color.

Cantaloupes

As juice and peeled and seeded fresh or frozen
Cantaloupes are a source of beta carotene, potassium, vitamin C, and folate.

Cantaloupe is a melon that is a good source of beta carotene and vitamin C, antioxidants that support the immune system and may help to prevent cancer and heart disease. It is also an excellent source of potassium, an electrolyte necessary to regulate the exchange of nutrients between cells and the fluid surrounding them. Muscle fatigue can sometimes be the result of low potassium stores.

Potassium can become depleted during vigorous exercise, diarrhea, or vomiting or in those taking diuretics that do not spare potassium. Major trauma to the body or prolonged stress can also trigger the release of hormones that deplete potassium. When you consume potassium, your body excretes sodium, and diets rich in potassium are associated with a decreased incidence of high blood pressure in those with salt-sensitive hypertension.

Cantaloupe also contains other unique compounds that are able to decrease the viscosity of the blood, thereby preventing the formation of blood clots in the cardiovascular system.

When adding fresh cantaloupe or other melons to smoothies, remove the rind and seeds and cut into chunks. Frozen melon can also be used.

Carrots

As fresh or bottled juice without added sodium
Carrot juice is an excellent source of vitamin C, vitamin B6, folate, beta carotene, magnesium, and potassium.

Carrot juice contains glutathione, a powerful antioxidant and anticarcinogen. Carrots also contain phthalides, compounds that regulate the manufacture of prostaglandin E2, a substance that increases the rate of cell division. Cells that divide rapidly are at greater risk for becoming cancerous. Carrot juice also contains plant estrogens that alleviate menopausal symptoms and help prevent breast cancer.

Carrots contain too much fiber and not enough juice to add them directly to a blender, so dust off your juicer and make some fresh carrot juice. Or you can purchase fresh carrot juice at your local market or health food store. Add carrot juice to any smoothie. Its sweet taste blends well with most fruit. Since the carotenes are fat soluble, you may want to add a teaspoon of flaxseed oil to the drink for better absorption or drink the smoothie with a fat-containing meal.

Cherries

Pitted fresh, dried, or frozen without added sugar
Cherries are a source of vitamin C, potassium, magnesium, and
phosphorus.

Cherries contain the reddish flavonoid pigment anthocyanin, which
together with vitamin C supports the growth of collagen, the protein
in connective tissue. This makes cherries a good food for those at risk
of developing osteoporosis or for those who put a great deal of wear
and tear on their connective tissue, such as athletes. Anthocyanins and
vitamin C also act to reduce inflammation and counter the effect of
histamines. Cherries are sources of compounds called salicylates, which
are a natural form of aspirin. Salicylates can also reduce inflammation.

Cherries have traditionally been used in the treatment of gout.

Pit fresh cherries before throwing them into the blender. Frozen
cherries are easily stored in the freezer.

Cranberries

As juice concentrate, fresh or frozen without added sugar, and
dried extract
Cranberries are a source of vitamin C and potassium.

Like all berries, these fruits are rich in anthocyanins and vitamin
C, two nutrients that support the growth of strong collagen fibers in the
soft connective tissue and bone. Cranberries are best known for their
ability to prevent bladder infections. This is due to the as yet unidentified "cranberry chemical" that prevents the adhesion of bacteria to the
wall of the bladder, making it easier for these pathogens to wash away in
the urine. Cranberries also contain salicylates, a natural form of aspirin,
which can reduce inflammation. Salicylates may also help to "thin" the
blood, preventing the formation of life-threatening blood clots.

Cranberry juice is very tart, so the bottled varieties are quite high
in sugar. To sweeten the tart cranberry, add bananas, molasses, honey,
or apple juice to a smoothie. When cranberries are in season, throw a
few bags in the freezer. Frozen whole cranberries add color and tart-
ness and are especially effective in sweet drinks. Dried cranberries can
be used to add color and texture to smoothies.

Dates

Whole pitted, chopped, and as date sugar (ground dried dates), preserved without sulfur

Dates are a source of calcium, magnesium, soluble and insoluble fiber, and folic acid.

Dates add fiber, folacin, and salicylates to fight cancer and heart disease, trace minerals and calcium for building bone density, and iron to prevent fatigue and menstrual problems.

Whole date puree is the easiest way to sweeten smoothies with dates. Purchase whole, pitted dates and puree them in a blender with water or add directly to smoothies. If they are very dry, soak them overnight.

Grapefruits

As juice, fresh, and bottled without added sugar

Grapefruits are a source of vitamin C, folate, magnesium, potassium, and inositol, a member of the vitamin B complex.

Grapefruit is the perfect fruit for those with heart disease. It contains the following: potassium, which lowers high blood pressure; pectin, a soluble fiber that lowers cholesterol levels in the blood; and vitamin C, which helps to stabilize unstable plaque lesions in arteries. Grapefruit also contains: flavonoids, terpenes, d-limonene, and coumarins, which prevent cancer; glutathione, the nutrient used by the liver for detoxification; and folate, which detoxifies homocysteine and prevents birth defects. Pink grapefruit is a source of two carotenes: beta carotene and beta-cryptoxanthin.

The flavonoid naringenin, found only in grapefruit, inhibits several liver enzymes responsible for drug metabolism. If you take calcium channel blockers, cyclosporin, or a benzodiazepine, check with your physician or pharmacist before adding grapefruit to your smoothies. Naringenin also prolongs the length of time caffeine remains in the blood, so less caffeine is necessary to produce alertness.

Fresh or bottled grapefruit sections add body and a tart flavor to smoothies.

Grapes

As juice, frozen concentrate, and seedless fresh, canned, or frozen
without added sugar
Grapes are a source of potassium and manganese.

Purple grapes contain a chemical called resveratrol, the same chemical
thought to be responsible for the protective effect of red wine on the
arteries of the heart. In two small studies of healthy subjects and rhesus
monkeys, Wisconsin researchers found that drinking three glasses of
purple grape juice a day reduced platelet aggregation by about 40 percent, making grape juice about as protective as daily aspirin for patients
with heart disease. Resveratrol also inhibits all three major stages of
cancer development: initiation, promotion, and progression.

Add bottled purple grape juice or whole seedless frozen or fresh
grapes to smoothies.

Kiwifruit

Kiwis are a source of vitamin C, potassium, and fiber.

Also called the Chinese gooseberry, this small, oval fruit has a fuzzy
surface and a distinctive green flesh studded with tiny purplish seeds. It
contains almost twice as much vitamin C (100 mg per fruit) as an
orange.

Baltimore researchers measured the effects of vitamins C and E
in twenty adults with normal blood cholesterol levels. Each participant
ate a 900-calorie meal that contained 50 percent saturated fat. Four
hours later, their arteries had widened by only 8 percent, about half as
much as they should have. When the participants, however, were given
800 units of vitamin E and 1,000 mg of vitamin C with the meal, the
blood vessels widened by 18 percent. This is the same dilation that was
measured when participants ate a zero-fat meal of the same calories.
These findings suggest that vitamins C and E may be able to counter-
act the effects of a high-fat meal.

To add kiwifruit to smoothies, cut the fruit into halves and scoop
out the flesh.

Mangoes

As juice, peeled fresh, and bottled without added sugar
Mangoes are a source of beta carotene, potassium, and
insoluble fiber.

This tropical fruit contains all the nutrients necessary for a healthy heart, low blood pressure, and a strong immune system.
Mango slices add a thick, smooth texture to smoothies.

Oranges

As juice, frozen juice concentrate, and peeled and seeded fresh,
frozen without added sugar, or canned
Oranges are a source of vitamin C, potassium, folic acid, phosphorus, magnesium, and pectin.

The folic acid in orange juice protects against birth defects and aids in the detoxification of homocysteine, a protein that is toxic to the arterial wall. It is packed with a variety of powerful antioxidants, including beta carotene, beta-cryptoxanthin, flavonoids, and terpenes, which strengthen the immune system and protect against colds and the flu. Pectin, the soluble fiber present in oranges, is associated with a decrease in cholesterol levels and may decrease the risk of cancer. Orange juice contains more glucose than other fruits and so is excellent to take when you need to raise blood glucose levels quickly. Concentrated orange juice adds sweetness and flavor to tofu, soy milk, milk, and protein mixes.

Papayas

As juice and peeled fresh, frozen, or bottled without added sugar
Papayas are a source of vitamin C, beta carotene, potassium, and
fiber.

The papaya fruit is a source of the unique protein-digesting enzyme papain, which is the enzyme used in commercial products as a meat tenderizer. Papain has anti-inflammatory properties and can be used as a digestive aid. In animal studies, papaya protected the stomach of lab animals from developing ulcers when the animals were fed aspirin and steroids. Both of these drugs are infamous for producing ulcers in humans.

Papaya is also a rich source of the antioxidant beta carotene, which the body converts to vitamin A, and potassium, which is needed to regulate blood pressure.

Papaya slices add a smooth thick texture to smoothies. If you wish to take advantage of the properties of papain, you must use either fresh or frozen papaya, since this enzyme is deactivated by the heat used in processing. Bottled papaya slices, however, are still rich in nutrients.

Peaches

Peeled and pitted fresh, dried, frozen without added sugar, or canned
Peaches are a source of beta carotene, vitamin C, potassium, and fiber.

Peaches are rich not only in the familiar beta carotene but also in zeaxanthin, another type of carotenoid with antioxidant properties. Both of these pigments are absorbed primarily by the ovaries and adipose tissue. The macula of the retina also absorbs zeaxanthin, where it protects the photoreceptor cells of the retina from free radicals generated by light.

Beta carotene is a source of the nontoxic provitamin A and together with vitamin C helps to prevent against infections, cancer, heart disease, and stroke. The fiber and potassium found in peaches decrease the high blood pressure found in hypertensives, and its plant estrogens can contribute to a decrease in menopausal symptoms. Dried peaches were found in one study to contain the most concentrated source of potassium.

To add dried peaches to smoothies, first soak peach slices in water or juice overnight, then puree. Then add the other smoothie ingredients. Frozen peaches are an easy way to add thickness to blender drinks. Canned peaches add a smooth texture to winter smoothies.

Pears

Peeled and cored fresh, frozen without added sugar,
    or canned
Pears are a source of fiber, potassium, vitamin C, B complex vitamins, manganese, and selenium.

Pears contain plant estrogens, which, along with the antioxidant and anticarcinogen glutathione, are recommended for the prevention of high blood pressure, stroke, and menopausal symptoms. Each pear contains folate, the B vitamin shown to prevent neural tube defects in infants. Folate is also involved with the detoxification of homocysteine, a protein that is toxic to the arterial cell wall and increases the risk of developing heart disease.

The flesh of the pear contains numerous gritty "stone" cells, which contain hemicellulose, a type of fiber that promotes the beneficial intestinal flora necessary for digestion and elimination in the colon. One pear contains a whopping five grams of fiber.

Canned pears blend well and add a thick texture and delicate sweetness to smoothies.

Pineapples

Peeled fresh or frozen without sugar
Pineapples are a source of vitamin C, potassium, manganese, and fiber.

Bromelain is a protein-digesting enzyme found only in fresh pineapple. It helps in the digestion of protein and is often used to improve nutrient absorption. Fresh pineapple juice when sipped acts as an anti-inflammatory that is useful when the throat is sore from an infection or irritation or inflamed from oral surgery.

This fruit is a good choice for those with heart disease. In the blood stream, bromelain decreases platelet aggregation, which reduces the risk of developing a life-threatening blood clot. Pineapple contains potassium, which increases the excretion of sodium and reduces blood pressure in those with hypertension.

Only fresh or frozen pineapple or pineapple juice contain bromelain, since the enzyme is destroyed by the heat of processing. Canned pineapple does not contain active enzymes. Pineapple juice is very sweet. Frozen pineapple and canned pineapple chunks add color and a mild flavor to smoothies.

Pumpkins

Canned puree without added sugar
Pumpkins are a source of provitamin A, potassium, and fiber.

Pumpkin contains two types of antioxidant carotenes: the more familiar beta carotene and the lesser known but more powerful alpha carotene. While beta carotene has demonstrated an ability to cause tumor regression and redifferentiation in some established cancers, alpha carotene's antitumor effect is up to ten times more effective. Both alpha and beta carotene are nontoxic precursors to vitamin A.

Canned pumpkin is heated during processing, and this will make the beta carotene contained in the pumpkin more absorbable.

Canned pureed pumpkin makes a healthful addition to any smoothie. It brings a thick, smooth texture and offers a change of pace from sweet fruits. Pumpkin puree works well with spicy flavorings such as ginger, cinnamon, nutmeg, and pumpkin pie spice.

Raspberries

Fresh or frozen without added sugar
Raspberries are a source of vitamin C, folic acid, potassium,
    calcium, magnesium, and insoluble fiber.

Raspberries are a great recovery food for athletes. They contain magnesium, potassium, and vitamin B6, all nutrients that are lost during vigorous exercise. Low potassium levels are often the cause of muscle weakness and cramps. Raspberries are also full of salicylates, natural compounds similar to aspirin that affect prostaglandin synthesis, reducing inflammation and pain.

Raspberries are also a good food for those at risk of heart disease. Salicylates help to prevent the formation of blood clots and have, at least by one researcher, been credited with the decrease in cardiovascular disease. Raspberries contain vitamin C, calcium, fiber, and anthocyanins, which are all linked to a decreased risk of developing heart disease. The polyphenols in berries show antiviral activity.

Fresh or frozen raspberries can be added to smoothies.

Strawberries

Hulled fresh or frozen without added sugar
Strawberries are a rich source of vitamin C, potassium, manganese, and biotin.

Strawberries have one of the highest antioxidant capacities of forty common fruits and vegetables. In a study of eight elderly women, a special beverage made from strawberry extract boosted the women's antioxidant capacity as much as by taking 1,250 mg of vitamin C.

Strawberries are also packed with health-giving phytochemicals, such as the following: polyphenols, compounds that may have antiviral activity; glutathione, a powerful detoxifier found in the liver; and salicylates, which help to thin the blood and reduce inflammation.

Fresh strawberries, when in season, add a fragrant note to smoothies. Frozen strawberries are available year-round and are a convenient way to add thickness and nutrient density to smoothies.

Tomatoes

As bottled low-sodium tomato juice, paste, or fresh juice
Tomato juice and paste are a source of vitamin B6, vitamin C, folate, beta carotene, potassium, and magnesium.

The red in tomato comes from the pigment lycopene, which is a powerful antioxidant from the carotene family. Lycopene enhances resistance to bacterial infections, may prevent prostate cancer, and may protect healthy cells from total body irradiation. Low levels of lycopene may increase an individual's risk for lung cancer. In a study of 93 patients with lung cancer and 102 control subjects who did not have the malignancy, the level of lycopene was significantly lower in the lung cancer group. The researchers also found that subjects with the lowest lycopene levels had a cancer risk three times that of subjects with the highest lycopene levels. In African-Americans, those with the lowest lycopene levels had an eightfold greater risk for cancer compared with those with the highest lycopene levels.

The folate found in tomatoes helps to detoxify homocysteine, a protein that damages the delicate walls of the artery. Folate also is needed by pregnant women to prevent neural tube defects in their offspring.

Tomato juice offers a change of pace from sweet smoothies. Tomato paste is a concentrated flavoring that works well with silken tofu, yogurt, and milks.

Watermelons

Peeled seedless fresh or frozen
Watermelons are a good source of potassium, lycopene, and
   vitamin C.

This melon is an excellent electrolyte replacer that is low in sugar and calories. It is one of the few dietary sources of lycopene, a pigment of the carotene family. A high dietary intake of the antioxidant lycopene is associated with a decrease in prostate and lung cancers. Smokers have low levels of this nutrient. Lycopene enhances resistance to bacterial infections and may protect healthy cells from total body irradiation.
Watermelon also contains vitamin C, the water-soluble vitamin that protects the watery areas of the cell from free radical damage and that is necessary for the manufacture of strong healthy connective tissue in muscle and bone. This fruit is another source of glutathione, a powerful antioxidant and anticarcinogen that also works with vitamin C to prevent cancer and heart disease.
Cut the watermelon into cubes when adding fresh melon to smoothies. Frozen watermelon can also be used.

HERBS

This is a very short list of some of the more common herbs added to smoothies; a complete list is beyond the scope of this book. We recommend that you purchase one of the excellent books on this subject listed in the appendix. Remember that herbs are powerful medicines and this power should be respected. Never take herbs without supervision if you are taking any other prescription drug. Never give herbs to children without the guidance of a health professional familiar with herbs. Never exceed the recommended dosage of an herb.

Astragalus

Astragalus membranaceus is a Chinese herb used as an immune stimulant, antioxidant, anti-inflammatory, and blood pressure regulator and to aid liver regeneration. Clinical trials have shown that the use of astragalus can reduce the incidence and shorten the course of the common cold and viral infections. It can be found as a component of liquid herbal extracts.

Echinacea

Echinacea is an American herb that comes from the purple coneflower plant. It contains a wide variety of phytochemicals that prevent infections, heal wounds, reduce the pain of arthritis, and may be useful in the treatment of cancer.

Echinacoside is the antibiotic component of this herb, which also has the ability to reduce inflammation such as that in arthritis. Echinacein is another substance found only in echinacea and prevents bacteria from invading tissues and is also able to stimulate faster wound healing.

Echinacea stimulates the production of interferon, T cells, and other white blood cells necessary for a strong immune system. Echinacea may also be useful in the treatment of cancer. Patients with inoperable liver cancer receiving toxic chemotherapies were treated with echinacea extract. After treatment with echinacea, the patients experienced a sharp reduction in chemotherapy-induced side effects, a greater quality of life, and a significant improvement in immune function. Echinacea that is part of a liquid herbal extract can be easily added to smoothies.

Ginger

Ginger root has been used as a digestive and circulatory stimulant for thousands of years. Recent research indicates that ginger acts much like aspirin, modifying the body's inflammatory response. This property has made it useful for the prevention of migraine headaches and in the treatment of other inflammatory conditions, including rheumatoid arthritis. Ginger is valuable for those at risk for heart disease. It contains antioxidants that protect the arterial walls, it reduces serum cholesterol levels, and it helps to prevent the formation of blood clots.

In controlled studies, ginger root was shown to be as effective as an over-the-counter drug in treating motion sickness. It also has been found useful in treating nausea and the morning sickness of early pregnancy. Add ginger root powder or fresh crushed ginger root to your smoothies.

Ginkgo

Ginkgo is made from the leaves of the *Ginkgo biloba* tree, one of the world's longest living tree species. In addition to a number of flavonoids, ginkgo is a also source of the unique ginkgolides.

These compounds stimulate the arterial cells to produce substances that prevent platelets from aggregating and forming blood clots. They also affect the tone of blood vessels, keeping the small arteries open and their muscle layers relaxed.

Ginkgo is used to enhance blood flow to the brain, reduce ringing in the ears (tinnitus) and to treat vascular diseases of the leg. Ginkgo is available as a tincture or as a liquid herbal extract.

Ginseng

Chinese or Korean ginseng (*Panax ginseng*) is a large, multibranched taproot that has been used by men in Asian cultures for centuries as a tonic, stimulant, and rejuvenator. With women it is used to relieve PMS and the hot flashes of menopause and to enhance sexual gland function and fertility. Today, it is often used to enhance athletic performance, to stimulate the immune system, and to aid in detoxification.

Ginseng's healing properties are believed to be due to a family of poorly understood chemicals called ginsenosides. Ginsenosides appear to prevent physical fatigue by enhancing the use of fatty acids for muscle fuel, prevent mental fatigue by balancing the hypothyroid-pituitary-adrenal axis, and even protect cells from radiation damage. You can add ginseng extract or liquid to smoothies.

Goldenseal

Goldenseal is an herb native to North America. Its active ingredients are believed to be berberine and hydrastine. Goldenseal is used in the treatment of bacterial, fungal, and protozoan infections. It appears to prevent the adhesion of some microbes to the host's cell wall preventing infection. Berberine also stimulates the immune system by activating macrophages, the white blood cells responsible for eating and destroying bacteria and viruses. Goldenseal may elevate blood pressure in some individuals and so it should not be used by those with high blood pressure, diabetes, glaucoma, or a history of stroke.

Goldenseal is often recommended to treat infectious diarrhea. Those traveling outside of the country may find this herb aids in the prevention of "travelers" diarrhea. It is also used to treat candida overgrowth and is recommended for those undergoing antibiotic therapy that can foster candida infections. Goldenseal is available as a tincture or as a liquid herbal extract.

Licorice

Licorice root is an herb that has been used for thousands of years in Eastern cultures. Its major active ingredient is glycyrrhizin, which breaks down into glycyrrhetinic acid, or GA. GA has anti-inflammatory properties that may aid in the relief of arthritis pain. It also inhibits liver damage due to chemical toxins and may reduce PMS symptoms by opposing estrogen and promoting progesterone. Glycyrrhizin mimics aldosterone, the hormone responsible for sodium balance in the body. In large doses it can elevate blood pressure and increase water retention, causing edema.

Licorice is traditionally used to treat stomach ulcers. In a twelve-week study of 874 people with duodenal ulcers, those treated with deglycerrhizinated licorice (to avoid edema and hypertension) had their ulcers heal faster than those given Tagamet, a commonly prescribed acid blocker. Some component other than GA increased prostaglandin production in the endothelial cells of the stomach. This protected the gastric mucosa from irritation.

Licorice is naturally very sweet. It is often used to mask the flavor of bitter herbs in liquid herbal extracts.

Milk Thistle

This herb comes from the seeds of the milk thistle plant. The main active component is silymarin. Silymarin is most often used to enhance liver function and to prevent damage to the liver by toxins and drugs. It is a more potent antioxidant than vitamin E.

Silymarin increases the amount of glutathione in the liver cell. Glutathione is responsible for the detoxification of a number of hormones, drugs, and chemicals.

Milk thistle seed is used to treat cirrhosis, chronic hepatitis, fatty liver, and psoriasis. It can be purchased as part of a liquid herbal extract.

Mint

Peppermint and spearmint are two varieties of mint—an ancient herb. The active ingredient is the aromatic oil. Spearmint contains carvone, and peppermint contains the more powerful menthol. Menthol soothes the digestive tract, relaxing the smooth muscle found there. It may help to prevent stomach ulcers and stimulate the secretion of bile.

When used fresh as a culinary herb, peppermint leaves are useful in preventing nausea and the morning sickness of pregnancy.

Tea

The tea tree is a small evergreen tree called *Camellia sinensis*. Green tea is simply the dried leaf of the bush, and black tea is the dried and then fermented leaf. Both black and green tea contain bioactive compounds.

Tea contains many powerful polyphenols. Catechins are found in green tea, and theaflavins and thearubigens are found in black tea. These antioxidants confer antiviral, antibacterial, and antifungal properties. They help prevent the development of cancer, inhibit the multiplication of viruses, and guard against food-borne pathogenic bacteria. Tea is good for the teeth. It is a natural source of fluoride, and its many antioxidants protect teeth from cavity-inducing bacteria.

Tea contains caffeine and theophylline, alkaloids that stimulate the brain, improving concentration and coordination. They are also natural diuretics, causing the kidneys to excrete more water. Caffeine acts as a natural painkiller and stimulant. A recent study found that green tea polyphenols increased the rate at which calories are burned 20–500 percent in a dose-dependent fashion, so tea drinking may be a useful part of a weight loss diet. Caffeine-free tea is available if you are sensitive to the effects of caffeine. Instant tea powder or green tea extract can also be added to smoothies.

Tea inhibits the absorption of iron from meat when taken at the same meal. This is a real plus for men and postmenopausal women for whom iron intake is linked to an increased risk of heart disease.

COMMON SUPPLEMENTS

The best source of vitamins, minerals, and other nutrients is found in fresh fruits and vegetables, whole grains, nuts and seeds, and dairy and animal products. Sometimes, however, we need more of a particular nutrient than we can get from our daily diet. Then we need to supplement our diet with isolated nutrients. Notice that I use the word *supplement*—never attempt to completely replace a needed nutrient. A poor diet with food supplements is still a poor diet. They cannot replace a healthy balanced whole foods diet.

Respect food supplements. Never take megadoses unless you are in the care of a knowledgable physician or nutritionist. Large amounts of some minerals can lower the blood levels of other minerals and some vitamins interfere with the action of prescription drugs.

Food supplements are available from a wide variety of sources. You can find them in health food stores or your local market in the health food section. If you have access to the Internet you can order almost any product and have it delivered within days. The Internet can boast of being the least expensive source of vitamins, minerals, and other health food products.

Acidophilus

Lactobacillus acidophilus and *Bifidobacterium bifidum* are healthful bacteria that live in the intestinal tract. There are many intestinal flora that live in symbiosis in the intestines, and they perform important functions, such as aiding the digestive processes. These healthy natural colonies are depleted when exposed to antibiotics, alcohol, and certain medications. When the healthy bacterium colonies are reduced, candida and other fungus then have room to grow, and candida infections result. Replenishing the micro flora with *Bifidobacterium bifidum* and *Lactobacillus acidophilus* is critical for proper immune function, cholesterol metabolism, and protection against cancer and for the elderly. Acidophilus should be added to all fruit drinks for those with candida. Mild-flavored powdered products are available that can be added to smoothies.

Arginine

Arginine is an amino acid that helps the smooth muscle cells in the arteries to relax. It is used in the treatment of high blood pressure, heart disease, and sexual dysfunction due to circulatory problems. Arginine may enhance the release of growth hormone.

You can purchase arginine in a powder form as arginine HCl or in combination with another amino acid, ornithine.

Brewer's Yeast

Yeast is a single-cell organism that multiplies rapidly within a matter of hours. Brewer's yeast is an excellent source of the B vitamins and chromium, the nutrients necessary for blood sugar regulation and energy production. This makes it the perfect supplement for diabetics and those with hypoglycemia. Brewer's yeast also contains the folate, magnesium, copper, selenium, and manganese needed to prevent and treat heart disease.

Calcium

Calcium is the macromineral that gives bone its hardness. Adequate calcium is necessary to prevent the thinning of the bone called osteoporosis. While almost all calcium is stored in the bones, teeth, and hard tissues, the one percent found in the soft tissues and extracellular fluid is very active metabolically. Here it works with magnesium to regulate heart beat, muscle contraction, and nerve conduction. Research has shown that supplemental calcium will lower elevated blood pressure in many instances.

Calcium and magnesium compete for absorption, so a high intake of one can lead to a deficiency in the other. Calcium is available by itself in a liquid and a powder form or as part of a calcium–magnesium supplement.

Creatine Monohydrate

Creatine is a nonstructural amino acid found in the muscle tissue, which is used in energy production. Athletes supplement creatine to increase muscle strength and build muscle size.

Lecithin

Lecithin is a dietary source of choline. Choline is a nutrient needed to produce acetylcholine, a neurotransmitter important for memory.

Choline is a component of cell membranes and of myelin, the insulating sheath around the nerves. Choline and lecithin have been shown to be essential for proper brain development in infants and children. Normally the body produces enough choline for neurotransmitter production, but when nerve cells are stressed the need for acetylcholine can outpace the rate of choline production. When this happens dietary lecithin can become an important source of the needed choline.

Lecithin is essential for proper liver function, and even a few weeks on a choline-free diet causes abnormalities in liver function. Choline supplementation reduces the urinary excretion of carnitine, an amino acid involved in energy production through the conservation of skeletal muscle carnitine. Large amounts of niacin taken to lower blood cholesterol levels may lower the amount of choline and lecithin available to the body. Lecithin must be present for choline synthesis.

Wheat germ and peanut butter are natural sources of lecithin. Lecithin granules suitable for smoothies can also be purchased. Lecithin is perishable and should be purchased fresh in an oxygen-free container.

Magnesium

Magnesium and calcium have similar functions and may oppose each other. For example, in muscle tissue, calcium stimulates contraction and magnesium relaxes it. This makes magnesium supplements useful in treating heart disease, high blood pressure, muscle cramps, and insomnia.

If you supplement your diet with large amounts of calcium you may create a magnesium deficiency, since both minerals must compete for the same receptors to be absorbed. Magnesium is available by itself in a liquid and a powder form or as part of a calcium–magnesium supplement.

Medium-Chain Triglycerides

Fat is a source of concentrated energy, but most fats take a long time to digest. When energy is needed immediately or when the digestive tract is unable to digest fats, medium chain triglyceride (MCT) oil may be your answer. Most of the fatty acids in food are long chain fatty acids, which must be digested in the small intestine and travel through the lymphvessels before reaching the bloodstream. MCTs do not need to be digested. They are short enough to enter the bloodstream whole, bypassing the lymphatic system. Add one tablespoon of MCT oil to a smoothie before an athletic event. If you have any kind of disease that causes malabsorption (newly diagnosed celiac disease, cancer, or AIDS), MCT oil can help you to regain lost weight. MCT oils can raise blood cholesterol levels, so if you use them regularly, have your cholesterol checked at your yearly physical. MCT oil is available at health food stores and pharmacies in a variety of flavors.

Tyrosine and Phenylalanine

Tyrosine and phenylalanine are amino acids necessary for the manufacture of epinephrine and norepinephrine, the neurotransmitters responsible for alertness and concentration. These nutrients can be added to smoothies as part of a protein supplement or separately in powder form.

Vitamin C

Vitamin C is a powerful antioxidant and is necessary for proper immune function. Antioxidants provide protection against toxins, pollution, secondhand smoke, and the effects of stress. It promotes wound healing and is necessary for tissue growth and repair, adrenal function, and healthy gums. Maintaining vitamin C levels also reduces cholesterol levels and high blood pressure and may help prevent atherosclerosis. Purchased in a powdered form, it is possible to measure small quantities to be added to smoothies. Buffered powder has magnesium, potassium, and calcium added to slow vitamin C's absorption, which allows the body to utilize more of the vitamin over a longer period of time.

OTHER INGREDIENTS

Caffeine

Caffeine is an alkaloid found naturally in tea, coffee, and cocoa and added frequently to soft drinks such as colas. It stimulates the cortex of the brain, improving concentration and coordination. Caffeine may also speed up metabolism, making it useful for weight loss.

High doses of caffeine may be useful in relieving muscle pain. University of Pittsburgh researchers measured pain in volunteers when the participants performed wrist curls after the blood was drained from their arms. The researchers found that pain was reported at double the level in those who received a placebo when compared to those who received a high dose of caffeine. Caffeine appears to work by blocking receptors for adenosine, a neurotransmitter thought to be involved in pain associated with decreased blood flow.

Carob

Carob is a natural flavoring agent that is similar in flavor to chocolate. It is used as a substitute for cocoa and chocolate, since it does not contain caffeine or theobromine, an alkaloid similar to caffeine. It contains protein, calcium, phosphorous, and some B vitamins.

Cocoa Powder

Cocoa is a lowfat source of chocolate flavor. Researchers have found that two tablespoons of cocoa contain 146 milligrams of flavonoid phenols (including resveratrol), potent natural antioxidants similar to those found in red wine (a five-ounce glass of red wine contains 210 mg of phenol). In the test tube, cocoa powder significantly inhibits the oxidation of LDL in vitro even better than red wine does. Cocoa contains caffeine and theobromine, mild natural stimulants, and phenylethylalamine, a chemical made naturally in the body when feeling in love and during the sexual act. Buy a high quality cocoa powder. Avoid cocoa mixes because they contain extra fat and sugar.

Coconut

Lowfat coconut milk adds tremendous flavor and the healthful omega-6 fatty acids without a lot of saturated fats. It is a source of concentrated calories. The coconut milk purchased in stores is actually coconut meat that is mixed with water, boiled, and strained. The reduced-fat versions have about one-quarter of the fat of regular coconut milk. Coconut extract can be used to add flavor and a sweet edge to smoothies without a lot of sugar. Shredded or grated coconut can also be added to smoothies. The mature coconut, about twelve inches (about 30 cm) long, is oval-shaped and has a thick, fibrous outer husk and a hard inner shell. The lining, or kernel, of the inner shell is a white, oily meat.

Flaxseed

Flaxseed is a source of the essential fatty acid linolenic acid, an omega-3 fatty acid that is the precursor to the series one prostaglandins. These prostaglandins act as vasodilators, antiplatelet aggregation agents, and anti-inflammatory factors. Flaxseeds also contain lignins, substances that act as antioxidants, help the body regulate hormone levels, and may inhibit tumor progression. Flaxseed is a source of both soluble and insoluble fiber and contains plant estrogens that relieve the symptoms of menopause. Add ground flaxseed powder or flaxseed oil to smoothies. All flax powders must be mixed with liquid.

Honey

Honey contains fructose and glucose, enzymes, and nominal amounts of vitamins and some trace minerals. Honey has natural antibiotic and sedative properties and has been used for centuries as a topical wound treatment. Researchers have found that those who use honey have fewer stomach ulcers than those who do not. Collected from flower nectar by bees, honey is actually sweeter than white sugar, and therefore it is possible to use less. Honey's color and flavor differs, depending on the type of flowers from which the bees collected pollen. This is why clover honey tastes so different from fireweed, strawberry, or rose

Warning

Children under the age of two years should never eat honey even if it is pasteurized. Honey can transmit heat-resistant botulism spores that can be very dangerous to children. Honey also can adversely affect blood sugar levels.

honey, for example. Add a teaspoon or two to sweeten sour and tart fruits, such as cranberries, lemons, grapefruit, and limes.

Molasses

Molasses is the nutrient-rich by-product of granulated table sugar production. It is a significant source of iron, calcium, potassium, thiamin, riboflavin, and niacin. One serving of molasses contains 3 mg of iron and 150 mg of calcium. Add a tablespoon as a sweetener for smoothies containing sour citrus fruits.

Peanut Butter

Peanuts are not really nuts but legumes. They are a source of protein, calcium, boron, vitamin E, folate, niacin, and heart-healthy monounsaturated fats. Peanuts contain resveratrol, the same substance behind red wine's ability to reduce heart disease, and salicylates, a natural form of aspirin. Peanut butter contains chromium and is a source of coenzyme Q10, which is necessary for energy production.

Add a few tablespoons of peanut butter to smoothies. Choose a natural-style peanut butter that has no added hydrogenated fat or salt.

Propolis

Propolis is a mixture of resins, vitamins, minerals, high amounts of bioflavonoids, and the antibacterial substance galangin, which is collected by bees from trees. Propolis helps sterilize the hive to inhibit the spread of bacteria, viruses, and fungi. It contains a natural antibiotic called galangin, which is purported to prevent low-grade infections and stimulate the immune system. Propolis is said to enhance the effectiveness of conventional antibiotics such as penicillin and streptomycin. Propolis can be found in your local health food store. Propolis is only available in its natural granules.

Psyllium Seed Powder

Psyllium seeds are rich sources of a soluble fiber called mucilage. The mucilage in psyllium seed aids in colon health. It prevents constipation and binds cholesterol and toxins in the intestine. When added to water, psyllium seed powder (also called ground psyllium seed) can swell to ten times its original size. It is odorless and bland in taste, but it has a gritty texture that is reduced by adding it to a drink containing a frozen fruit. Start with one teaspoon of psyllium powder and gradually work up to one tablespoon, to avoid developing gas.

Pumpkin Seeds

Pumpkin seeds contain protein, iron, and heart-healthy mono-unsaturated fats. They also contain alanine, glutamic acid, and glycine, the amino acids used to treat prostate enlargement. Ground pumpkin seeds (pumpkin seed butter) can be added to smoothies to increase their fat content.

Sea Vegetables

Algae

Algae such as spirulina, blue-green algae, and chlorella are grown, harvested, dried, and then sold for their supplemental protein, vitamin, and mineral content. They are rich sources of the trace minerals. Chlorella and spirulina provide the antimutagen pigment chlorophyll as well as beta carotene, RNA, and superoxide dismutase. Algae tends to be easily digested and assimilated and is a good alternative for those who have a hard time taking regular vitamin pills. Powdered algae is easy to add to smoothies but does add a mild seaweed flavor, which can be masked with flavoring, sweetener, or spices.

Kelp

This sea vegetable contains easily assimilated forms of minerals. This is particularly beneficial for those with mineral deficiencies from long-term dieting or fast-food meals. Kelp can be purchased dried, granulated, or powdered and can be added in small quantities to smoothies.

Sesame Seeds

Sesame seeds are rich in substances called lignins. Lignins act as protectors against hormonally related cancers, through their estrogenic activity, and they may inhibit tumor progression. Sesame seeds contain: diosgenin, a phytochemical shown to prevent cancer cells from multiplying; beta-sitosterol, gamma-sitosterol, and stigmasterol, phytochemicals that inhibit the uptake of cholesterol from foods in the diet; and coenzyme Q10, the enzyme necessary in energy production. Sesame seeds are also high in fiber and oil, both of which delay gastric emptying so that more minerals can be absorbed.

Add sesame seed meal or ground sesame seeds (also called tahini) to your smoothie for a mineral boost.

Stevia

Stevia is a natural, sweet-tasting plant extract that contains no calories and is an ideal sweetener for diabetics and hypoglycemics. It is one of the few sweeteners available that does not appear to raise blood sugar levels. Some researchers believe it has the potential for inhibiting fat absorption and decreasing hypertension. Stevia is available in liquid or powdered form.

Sunflower Seeds

Sunflower seeds are sources of protein, thiamin, vitamin B6, vitamin E, potassium, and iron. Ground sunflower seeds or sunflower seed butter add a fresh nutty taste to smoothies.

Wheat Germ

Wheat germ is the nutrient-dense embryo of the wheat berry. It contains copper, manganese, some B vitamins, and octacosanol and is one of the richest natural sources of vitamin E and insoluble fiber.

In the ongoing study of 44,000 American male health professionals, Boston researchers found that men who ate twenty-five grams or more of fiber-rich food each day were 55 percent less likely to suffer a fatal myocardial infarction than men who ate twelve grams of fiber or less. One tablespoon of wheat germ will add two grams of protein and one gram of fiber to your smoothie.

PROTEIN SOURCES

Protein exists in all living cells and is necessary for tissue and cell regeneration, enzyme and hormone production, building and repairing muscle tissue, and increasing nitrogen retention at the cellular level.

Protein Powder

Protein powders offer the opportunity for your body to get all the nourishment it needs without the saturated fat that accompanies animal protein sources. When added to smoothies, protein balances out the carbohydrates present from added sweeteners and fruit. It helps to prevent the body from producing too much insulin and keeps the glucose levels even, so that you do not experience the fatiguing symptoms of low blood sugar.

Protein powder can be made from cow's milk, goat's milk, eggs, soybeans, and other plant sources and can be supplemented with a variety of vitamins, minerals, fatty acids, and carbohydrates. It is available in a wide variety of flavors including vanilla, chocolate, and strawberry. Read the label of any protein supplement carefully before you buy, to be sure that it is suitable for your needs. *Protein powders are not substitutes for infant formula and should never be given to infants.*

Do not confuse protein supplements with powered milk replacements. Some formulas are designed to taste or function like dairy milk but do not contain the same amounts of protein, calcium, vitamin D, or riboflavin as does milk. We found a tasty soy-based tofu powder that was less grainy than regular soy powders. It was fortified with calcium and tasted like milk, but a look at the label revealed the protein content to be only one gram per tablespoon, compared to five grams of protein for most soy protein.

Always read the label. A protein supplement that is suitable for competitive athletes is often not the best choice for a person recovering from illness or one looking to lose weight (although some work very well for these purposes). Do not hesitate to ask the salesperson to identify each ingredient and explain why it is present in the formula.

Hydroyslate protein has been partially broken down (digested) into smaller protein fragments so that the body's immune system cannot recognize its source and mount an immune reaction (allergy). If you suspect you have a food allergy, a hydroyslate protein supplement may be a good choice. The more a protein is digested, however, the more unpalatable its taste.

Egg White Powder

Egg whites contain all of the essential amino acids without the cholesterol and fat that a whole egg contains. Dehydrated egg white is often used to increase the protein content of protein powders. Raw egg whites may be contaminated with bacteria and should never be added to drinks.

Cow's Milk

Each eight-ounce glass of milk provides eight grams of protein in the form of casein and whey.

Milk is also a source of calcium, magnesium, potassium, vitamin D, and riboflavin. Avoid whole milk, since it is a source of saturated fat and cholesterol. Choose nonfat plain milk, acidophilus milk, or buttermilk for your smoothies. Nonfat cottage cheese adds a thick texture without fat.

Goat's Milk

Goat's milk is available in the dairy case of many grocery stores and health food stores. As an alternative to cow's milk, it may be helpful to those with dairy allergies. However, it does contain lactose, the milk sugar many people cannot digest, and milk fat, which is associated with heart disease.

Soy

Soy foods are excellent sources of vegetable protein as well as numerous phytochemicals, including: antioxidants, which prevent free radical damage; lignins, which inhibit tumor progression; phytoestrogens, which protect against hormone-related cancers and reduce menopausal symptoms; and sitosterols, which mimic cholesterol and prevent its reabsorption in the intestine. Soy foods also contain calcium and essential fatty acids, are cholesterol-free, and are low in sodium and total fat.

Soy foods that can be added to smoothies are soy milk, tofu, mild white miso (for vegetable-based smoothies), and protein powders that contain soy protein isolates.

Soy Milk

Soy milk is made by boiling ground whole soybeans in water and separating the liquid from the fiber. It contains no cholesterol or saturated fat. Soy milk is the vegan choice for those who would like to avoid lactose, the milk sugar that thirty to fifty million Americans are unable to digest. With soy milk, it is possible to avoid the hormones and antibiotics that are now used to produce dairy milk.

Soy milk is available in full-fat (2 percent), lowfat (1 percent), and nonfat versions. Full-fat soy milk is a good choice for meal replacement smoothies. The soy oil provides essential fatty acids, increases the absorption of fat-soluble vitamins, helps to keep blood glucose levels even, and decreases the appetite. Nonfat soy milk adds protein and soy phytochemicals to smoothies for a quick pick-me-up.

Soy milk is available in a variety of forms. Some are plain with no flavoring or added sweeteners. Some are flavored with cocoa, carob, vanilla, cinnamon, or almond, with brown rice syrup or malted barley added for sweetness and sea salt, canola oil, and soy protein added to increase flavor and texture. Fresh soy milk (sold in the dairy case) usually has a milder taste than does packaged.

For most folks, soy milk is an acquired taste. Shop around until you find a brand that suits your taste buds, since flavor and texture vary widely from brand to brand. For smoothies, we recommend that you choose a flavored soy milk that is fortified with calcium, vitamin D, and riboflavin.

Tofu

Tofu is made by curdling fresh, hot soy milk in a process similar to making cottage cheese. The curds are then pressed together to give the consistency of soft cheese. Tofu is available in textures ranging from extra firm to soft and silken. For smoothies, choose soft or silken tofu. Tofu adds body and creaminess to smoothies and takes on whatever flavor is added to the drink. Full-fat tofu is a good choice for meal replacement smoothies, since it contains the heart-healthy omega-3 fatty acids. Like soy milk, the flavor of tofu varies with the brand. Fresh, refrigerated tofu often has a less beany taste than do aseptic packaged varieties.

Yogurt

Yogurt is an excellent source of calcium, magnesium, zinc, riboflavin, and protein. It is naturally rich in healthful bacteria, such as *Lactobacillus bulgaricus, Lactobacillus acidophilus,* and *Streptococcus thermophilus.* These bacteria promote the regrowth of the healthy microflora in the gut after they have been killed by antibiotics, preventing diarrhea. Yogurt contains antibiotic substances. It prevents the development of vaginal infections, stimulates the immune system by increasing the level of interferon, and stimulates natural killer-cell activity. Those who cannot digest other dairy products generally tolerate yogurt. Use only nonfat yogurt with no artificial sweeteners that contains live cultures. This will be marked on the label; look for it. Flavored yogurts are an easy way to add extra fruit flavors to smoothies. Frozen yogurt can also be used in smoothies, but since it lacks live cultures it does not have the same nutritional properties. Consider frozen yogurt a flavor of ice cream.

PURCHASING TIPS

Buy organic produce whenever possible. Organic produce is grown without pesticides or herbicides. These chemicals can suppress the immune system, and many are suspected of causing cancer.

Buy produce that is local and in season. Produce that is shipped long distances must be picked before it is ripe and will be less sweet and have less overall flavor.

Buy ripe fruits, as they are softer, sweeter, easier to digest, and have higher nutritional value. Fruits smell sweet when they are ripe. Generally, smell a fruit near the stem to check for ripeness.

Avoid produce with mold and discard any fruit that becomes moldy. Berries are especially fragile.

Frozen fruit is the next best thing to fresh. Many berries and tropical fruits may be available in your area only in the freezer section

of your local grocery. Sometimes frozen fruits are even pre-
ferred, because they add a creamy, ice cream–like texture to
smoothies. Buy only fruit that is frozen without added sugar
or juice.

Canned fruit can be used in place of fresh and offers the conve-
nience of easy storage. For example, canned peaches and apricots are widely available, and a variety of canned fruits can be
found in single-serving containers. They are soft and blend well
without slicing and add a rich creamy texture to smoothies. We
recommend purchasing fruit canned in fruit juice or light syrup.
Heavy syrup contains an amazing amount of sugar and should
be avoided. The fruit juice can be added to the blender with its
fruit or refrigerated and added to another smoothie. However,
to reduce the sugar and calorie content of a smoothie, drain the
juice/syrup before adding the fruit to smoothies. For a thicker
smoothie, you can freeze these serving-size cups of canned fruit.
Canned vegetables can also be used. Pumpkin puree adds a con-
siderable amount of beta carotene and fiber and makes a great
fall treat.

STORAGE TIPS

Smoothies made with ice should be drunk immediately. All other
smoothies can be stored in the refrigerator for up to twenty-four
hours.

To revive a stored smoothie: Pour the smoothie into a blender with
1/4 cup ice and blend until smooth.

Leftover smoothies? Make smoothie pops. Pour unused smoothies
into ice pop molds and store in the freezer for quick snacks.

Rice milk, soy milk, and almond milk can all be purchased in aseptic packages, which last for up to a year unopened. Keep unopened containers in the pantry so you'll have some on hand
when you don't have time to shop.

Oat Milk

This is a tasty alternative to dairy milk. It adds a creamy texture and soluble fiber to smoothies. This recipe makes one serving.

1 cup rolled oats or oat bran
1 cup filtered water

Place the oats and water into a blender and process until the water is cream colored. Pour the mixture into another container and rinse the blender container. Strain the mixture through a tea strainer or cheesecloth, return the oat milk to the blender, and add smoothie ingredients. Store any unused portion covered in the refrigerator. It is best if used within two days.

If you desire a smoothie with a higher fiber content, add the smoothie ingredients directly to the blender after mixing the oats and milk.

Calories	156	Protein	7 g
Calories from fat	23	Fiber	4 g
Total fat	3 g	Magnesium	62 mg
Carbohydrates	27 g	Thiamin	0.3 g

Seed or Nut Milk

Although almonds are the most popular, sesame or sunflower seeds, filberts (hazelnuts), cashews, or any other raw seeds or nuts can be used to make nut or seed milks.

1/2 cup fresh whole nuts or seeds of choice
1 cup filtered water
Sweetener (2 to 3 dates, 1 tablespoon raisins,
  or 1 teaspoon honey)

In a small bowl combine the nuts or seeds, sweetener, and water. Cover and let soak overnight.

Pour the mixture into a blender and process until the mixture is creamy. Pour the mixture into another container and rinse the blender container. Strain the mixture through a tea strainer or cheesecloth, return it to the blender, and add smoothie ingredients. Store any unused portion covered in the refrigerator. It is best if used within two days.

Calories	52	Carbohydrates	13 g
Calories from fat	3	Protein	54 g
Total fat	0 g	Fiber	0 g

Rice Milk

This is a lowfat, creamy alternative to dairy milk. This recipe works well with any cooked grain, including wheat, oats, rye, quinoa, and barley. It makes about one serving.

1/4 cup cooked grains, such as brown rice
1 cup filtered water

Place the cooked grains and water into a blender and process until the water is creamy. Pour the mixture into another container and rinse the blender container. Strain the mixture through a tea strainer or cheesecloth. Store any unused portion covered in the refrigerator. It is best if used within two days.

Calories	52	Carbohydrates	13 g
Calories from fat	3	Protein	54 g
Total fat	0 g	Fiber	0 g

CHAPTER 2

Just for the Taste of It

*H*ere are some of our favorite taste delights.

Fruit Shake

This has to be our favorite all-around recipe. Milk and banana are both mild in flavor and work well with any fruit.

1 cup milk of choice

1 frozen banana, cut into pieces

1/2 cup fruit of choice

Calories	214	Calcium	319 mg
Calories from fat	12	Magnesium	69 mg
Total fat	1 g	Riboflavin	1 mg
Carbohydrates	44 g	Vitamin B12	1 mcg
Protein	10 g	Vitamin B6	1 mg
Fiber	5 g		

Daiquiri

Here's a refreshing, light smoothie for those very hot days of summer.

2 cups ice

1 orange, peeled and seeded

1 tangerine, peeled and seeded

1/2 grapefruit, peeled and seeded

1 tablespoon lime juice

1 tablespoon sweetener, optional

Calories	141	Magnesium	38 mg
Calories from fat	5	Potassium	555 mg
Total fat	1 g	Folic acid	70 mcg
Carbohydrates	36 g	Vitamin C	141 mg
Protein	3 g	Vitamin A	119 mcg
Fiber	6 g		

Peaches and Cream

This makes a healthy summer drink. In the winter, substitute vanilla yogurt for the frozen.

1 cup lowfat frozen yogurt, flavor of choice

1 cup peach slices, fresh or frozen

About 200 mg vitamin C powder

Calories	312	Fiber	3 g
Calories from fat	20	Calcium	130 mg
Total fat	2 g	Potassium	653 mg
Carbohydrates	65 g	Riboflavin	0.4 mg
Protein	7 g	Vitamin C	211 mg

Orange Crush

Blend the first three ingredients, then add the sparkling water. Blend briefly, just enough to mix the ingredients.

1 cup orange sorbet

1 orange, peeled and seeded

about 200 mg vitamin C powder

1 cup sparkling mineral water

Calories	312	Protein	2 g
Calories from fat	2	Fiber	3 g
Total fat	0 g	Vitamin C	272 mg
Carbohydrates	78 g		

Cherry Cheesecake

When the urge for cheesecake hits, try this lowfat, high-flavor alternative.

1 1/2 cups frozen cherries, pitted

1 cup nonfat cottage cheese

1/2 cup nonfat milk

Calories	359	Fiber	5 g
Calories from fat	21	Calcium	344 mg
Total fat	2 g	Potassium	691 mg
Carbohydrates	48 g	Riboflavin	0.3 mg
Protein	37 g	Vitamin A	200 mcg

Citrus Light

Here's an unusual treat that is not overwhelmingly sweet.

1 1/2 cups watermelon pieces, seedless

1 orange, peeled and seeded

1/2 cup lime sorbet

1/4 lemon, peeled and seeded

Calories	272	Fiber	5 g
Calories from fat	12	Potassium	557 mg
Total fat	1 g	Thiamin	0.3 mg
Carbohydrates	66 g	Vitamin B6	0.5 mg
Protein	3 g	Folic acid	47 mcg

Kevin's Orange Sherbet Cup

This smoothie tastes like a creamsicle in a glass. It's a great way to "hide" soy milk in children's drinks. Just a reminder: *Never* add herbs or food supplements to smoothies for children without checking with your pediatrician for dosages.

1 cup milk of choice

1/2 cup orange sherbet

1 teaspoon lecithin granules

1/2 teaspoon pure vanilla extract, optional

Calories	230	Fiber	0 g
Calories from fat	53	Calcium	322 mg
Total fat	6 g	Potassium	406 mg
Carbohydrates	36 g	Vitamin B12	1 mcg
Protein	9 g		

Fruit Salad

This recipe provides three of the recommended five daily servings of fruits and vegetables.

1 cup strawberries

1/2 cup ice

1 navel orange, peeled and seeded

1/2 lemon, peeled and seeded

1/4 grapefruit, peeled and seeded

Calories	135	Fiber	8 g
Calories from fat	8	Potassium	608 mg
Total fat	1 g	Folic acid	75 mcg
Carbohydrates	33 g	Vitamin C	190 mg
Protein	3 g		

Chocolate Fix

For those days when you have to have chocolate, this protein-rich smoothie is a great meal replacement.

1 cup soy milk

1/2 cup chocolate lowfat frozen yogurt

4 ounces soft or silken tofu

2 tablespoons vanilla or chocolate protein powder

Calories	431	Calcium	356 mg
Calories from fat	145	Magnesium	170 mg
Total fat	16 g	Zinc	3 mg
Carbohydrates	32 g	Riboflavin	0.5 mg
Protein	45 g	Thiamin	1 mg
Fiber	6 g		

Summertime Punch

Here's the perfect recipe to make in large batches. Serve this at brunches or backyard barbecues.

1 part purple grape juice

1 part frozen red seedless grapes

1 part watermelon pieces, seedless

1 part cantaloupe pieces

Calories	189	Potassium	658 mg
Calories from fat	10	Niacin	1 mg
Total fat	1 g	Vitamin B6	0.4 mg
Carbohydrates	46 g	Vitamin A	295 mcg
Protein	2 g	Beta carotene	2661 mcg
Fiber	2 g		

Nutmeg Shake

This is Maureen's favorite drink. The banana disguises the gritty texture of soy protein.

10 ounces nonfat milk

1 banana

2 tablespoons vanilla soy protein powder

1 teaspoon ground nutmeg

Calories	292	Calcium	442 mg
Calories from fat	23	Magnesium	75 mg
Total fat	2.5 g	Potassium	967 mg
Carbohydrates	43 g	Riboflavin	1 mg
Protein	29 g	Vitamin B12	1 mcg
Fiber	3 g		

Cherry Coconut

Increase the mineral content of this smoothie by adding a powdered calcium-magnesium supplement.

1 1/2 cups frozen cherries

1/2 cup vanilla lowfat yogurt

1/2 cup lowfat coconut milk

2 tablespoons shredded coconut

1 teaspoon coconut extract

Calories	432	Fiber	6 g
Calories from fat	160	Iron	3 mg
Total fat	18 g	Magnesium	101 mg
Carbohydrates	60 g	Potassium	1029 mg
Protein	10 g	Zinc	2 mg

Banana Cream

This smoothie is like a slice of banana and coconut cream pie in a glass. Add a scoop of protein and a calcium-magnesium powder to this recipe for a nutrition boost.

1/2 cup lowfat coconut milk

1/2 cup nonfat milk

1 1/2 frozen bananas, cut into pieces

1 teaspoon coconut extract

Calories	319	Iron	3 mg
Calories from fat	99	Magnesium	116 mg
Total fat	11 g	Potassium	1132 mg
Carbohydrates	49 g	Vitamin B6	1 mg
Protein	7 g	Folic acid	55 mcg
Fiber	4 g		

CHAPTER 3

Energizers

Smoothies to Beat Fatigue

E nergy levels can drop when you are stressed, you are becoming ill, or you are just getting over an illness. Even when you are healthy, your energy levels can flag. These smoothies are designed to help get you up and moving.

Sleepy brains can be the result of serotonin production in the brain. In general, protein-rich foods stimulate the brain, while carbohydrate-rich foods make the brain more sleepy. By adding protein-containing ingredients to a smoothie while minimizing carbohydrates, you can affect which neurotransmitters are produced in your brain.

Sometimes you find that your brain is willing but the flesh is weak. Muscles rely on glucose for fuel. When something goes wrong with fuel delivery, an energy shortage results. The proper nutrients will assure that sufficient energy is available at the right time.

GENERAL DIETARY RECOMMENDATIONS

Eat breakfast. After its overnight fast, your body needs nourishment to start the day. If you skip breakfast, your blood sugar

levels will fall before lunch, leaving your limbs sleepy and your
brain foggy.

Have a high-protein snack at midmorning. Even a little protein
provides the brain with ample amounts of the amino acid tyrosine. This is the neurotransmitter that stimulates your brain.

Be aware that fatigue can be caused by food allergies. The most
common food allergens are milk, wheat, and corn. Fortified
soy milk is a superior substitute for cow's milk.

Be careful when you eat carbohydrates. Carbohydrates promote
the synthesis of serotonin, the neurotransmitter that quiets you
down. Avoid eating simple carbohydrates by themselves, since
they can make you sleepy.

SMOOTHIE INGREDIENTS TO INCREASE ENERGY

Brewer's Yeast

Brewer's yeast is a rich source of all the B vitamins including folic acid
and pyroxidine. The B vitamins are necessary to release energy from
carbohydrates. Pyridoxine (B6) is associated with a vast number of
enzymes, particularly those involving amino acids. It is essential for the
synthesis of the neurotransmitters serotonin, dopamine, and noradren-
aline. A vitamin B6 deficiency may result in low blood levels of vitamin
C, increased excretion of calcium, zinc, and magnesium, and reduced
copper absorption. Folic acid is also involved in the production of
dopamine, the "feel good" neurotransmitter.

Caffeine

Caffeine is a natural stimulant. The amount of caffeine found in coffee
is 100 to 200 mg per cup. One cup of coffee is sufficient to provide
enough caffeine to increase concentration, reaction time, and mental
alertness. The amount of caffeine found in tea is 40 to 80 mg per cup.

Creatine

Creatine is manufactured in the body from the amino acids arginine,
glycine, and methionine. Research suggests that reduced levels of muscle
creatine may impair muscle cell metabolism and protein synthesis, and

lower-than-normal levels of creatine have been found in patients with muscle disease, fibromyalgia, and rheumatoid arthritis. Creatine powder has a bland taste and can be purchased in health food stores. Smaller doses (one to three grams) are just as good (and perhaps safer) than is short-term use of larger doses (fifteen to thirty grams).

Iron

Fatigue is one of the most noticeable symptoms of iron deficiency anemia. Iron deficiency is common in growing children and women of childbearing years. Sources of iron include: sea vegetables such as spirulina, dulse, and algae; dried fruit such as raisins and prunes; brewer's and nutritional yeast; wheat germ and bran; and molasses, sunflower seed butter, and tofu.

Magnesium

This mineral is an essential part of hundreds of enzyme systems that support normal energy levels. It is necessary for proper nerve and muscle function. Magnesium deficiency causes fatigue and muscle weakness. Magnesium is available as a liquid in health food stores. Or, you can add bananas, blueberries, carrot juice, cherries, dates, grapefruits, oranges, tomato juice, and raspberries to increase the magnesium content of your smoothies.

Medium Chain Triglycerides

Fat is a source of concentrated energy, but most fats take a long time to digest. When energy is needed immediately or when the digestive tract is unable to digest fats, medium chain triglyceride (MCT) oil may be your answer. This oil provides a type of fatty acid that does not need to be digested before it is absorbed. MCTs enter the bloodstream whole, bypassing the lymphatic system. Many athletes add MCT oil to their drinks as a ready source of concentrated energy. However, there are some indications that MCTs reduce the secretion of growth hormone in the brain. This hormone is necessary for tissue repair. Too much MCT may therefore delay healing of tendon and muscle injuries. Check with your nutritionist or coach before adding MCT to your smoothies.

Lack of Energy from Heart Problems

Coenzyme Q10 allows the cell to burn fatty acids for fuel more efficiently, and the amino acid carnitine allows more effective use of the limited oxgen supply. Increasing your intake of these nutrients will increase energy production in your heart muscle. Both of these supplements can be purchased as part of a protein powder.

If you have any kind of disease that causes malabsorption (newly diagnosed celiac disease, cancer, or AIDS), MCT oil can help you to regain lost weight.

MCT oil is available at health food stores and pharmacies in a variety of flavors.

Nut Butters

The fiber and fat found in nut butters (ground nuts) increase the time a meal spends in the stomach, slowing the release of glucose into the blood, which prevents hypoglycemia. Nuts also contain folic acid, B vitamins, magnesium, potassium, and small quantities of zinc. A deficiency of any one of these nutrients can cause fatigue. Almond butter, cashew butter, and peanut butter are some nut butters that can be added to smoothies.

Potassium

This electrolyte (together with sodium) is responsible for the generation of electrical potential that causes muscle contraction and heartbeat. All fruits and most vegetables are excellent sources of potassium.

Protein

As little as two ounces of protein contains enough of the amino acid tyrosine to stimulate the production of the alertness neurotransmitters dopamine and norepinephrine. When your brain is producing dopamine and norepinephrine, you feel up, active, and motivated. Protein foods also delay the amount of time food spends in the stomach. This means that carbohydrates present in the meal are released slowly into the bloodstream, avoiding sugar highs and lows. Lack of protein is often the cause of midmorning slump. Good sources of proteins include milk, soy foods, and protein powders.

Tyrosine

Tyrosine is an amino acid that is converted by the body into epinephrine and norepinephrine, the neurotransmitters used by brain cells to promote alertness and concentration. Tyrosine can be purchased in powdered form and added to smoothies. Extra tyrosine is often added to nutritional supplements.

Mocha Magic

This smoothie is a healthier alternative to coffee. The protein and caffeine in this drink will give your brain the boost it needs to keep working.

10 ounces milk of choice

1 frozen banana, cut into pieces

2 to 3 tablespoons cocoa powder

2 tablespoons protein powder

1 to 2 tablespoons instant coffee powder

Calories	334	Calcium	459 mg
Calories from fat	28	Iron	2 mg
Total fat	3 g	Magnesium	139 mg
Carbohydrates	49 g	Potassium	1303 mg
Protein	32 g	Zinc	2 mg
Fiber	3 g	Riboflavin	1 mg

The Energizer

Need energy but have no time for a full meal? This smoothie has all the B vitamins and protein you need to stimulate the production of the alertness neurotransmitters.

1 cup vanilla whole soy milk

1 frozen banana, cut into pieces

1 tablespoon vanilla protein powder

1 teaspoon brewer's yeast

1 to 3 teaspoons MCT oil

Liquid ginseng supplement (see label for
   recommended dosage)

Calories	324	Fiber	7 g
Calories from fat	69	Vitamin B12	3 mcg
Total fat	8 g	Folic acid	160 mcg
Carbohydrates	50 g	Beta carotene	984 mcg
Protein	17 g	Vitamin E	7 mg

Grapefruit Tea

Here's a summer alternative to hot tea or coffee. This smoothie contains a small amount of caffeine to boost your energy levels and mental awareness. The grapefruit prevents the breakdown of caffeine, so it remains effective longer. Serve this smoothie along with a protein-containing meal, to keep you alert and awake.

1 cup brewed green or black tea, cooled

1 cup grapefruit pieces

2 to 3 ice cubes

Calories	91	Protein	1 g
Calories from fat	2	Fiber	1 g
Total fat	0 g	Iron	1 mg
Carbohydrates	23 g	Potassium	410 mg

Apple Kick

The protein and ginseng in this drink stimulate your brain, while the magnesium and calcium provide the nutrients needed for proper nerve and muscle function.

1 cup nonfat yogurt, flavor of choice

1/4 cup apple juice concentrate

6 ice cubes

Liquid magnesium supplement (see label for
  recommended dosage)

Flavored liquid ginseng supplement (see label for
  recommended dosage)

Calories	243	Calcium	470 mg
Calories from fat	6	Potassium	892 mg
Total fat	1 g	Zinc	2 mg
Carbohydrates	46 g	Riboflavin	1 mg
Protein	13 g	Vitamin B12	1 mcg
Fiber	0 g		

Chocolate Jolt

This is a great light-tasting drink for athletes or those who need a quick jolt of energy.

1 cup almond milk

1 frozen banana, cut into pieces

3 tablespoons (or to taste) cocoa powder

2 tablespoons protein powder

1 to 3 teaspoons MCT oil

Calories	537	Magnesium	249 mg
Calories from fat	284	Zinc	3 mg
Total fat	32 g	Riboflavin	1 mg
Carbohydrates	38 g	Niacin	3 mg
Protein	31 g	Vitamin E	11 mg
Fiber	3 g		

Green Genie

This recipe provides calcium, magnesium, creatine, and malic acid, nutrients that may help to provide relief for those with fibromyalgia, chronic fatigue, or other types of muscle fatigue. The chlorophyll supplement makes it green.

1 cup apple juice

1/2 cup plain nonfat yogurt

4 ice cubes

2 tablespoons lemon juice

1 to 3 grams creatine powder (see label for recommended dosage)

1 teaspoon liquid chlorophyll

Calories	189	Calcium	248 mg
Calories from fat	5	Iron	1 mg
Total fat	1 g	Potassium	623 mg
Carbohydrates	40 g	Zinc	1 mg
Protein	7 g	Vitamin B12	1 mcg
Fiber	0 g		

Cherry Jolt

Enjoy this quick energy-rich meal replacement.

1 cup frozen cherries

1/2 cup calcium-fortified orange juice

2 tablespoons protein powder

1 to 3 teaspoons MCT oil

1 teaspoon brewer's yeast

Calories	273	Calcium	231 mg
Calories from fat	57	Iron	1 mg
Total fat	6 g	Niacin	2 mg
Carbohydrates	38 g	Thiamin	1 mg
Protein	21 g	Folic acid	164 mcg
Fiber	4 g		

Berry Wake-Up

The protein, fat, and fiber in this drink will help to prevent the low blood sugar that often occurs in the afternoon.

1 cup berry nonfat yogurt

1 cup frozen strawberries

2 tablespoons almond butter

Calories	427	Calcium	457 mg
Calories from fat	183	Iron	2 mg
Total fat	20 g	Magnesium	145 mg
Carbohydrates	51 g	Zinc	3 mg
Protein	16 g	Vitamin E	7 mg
Fiber	5 g		

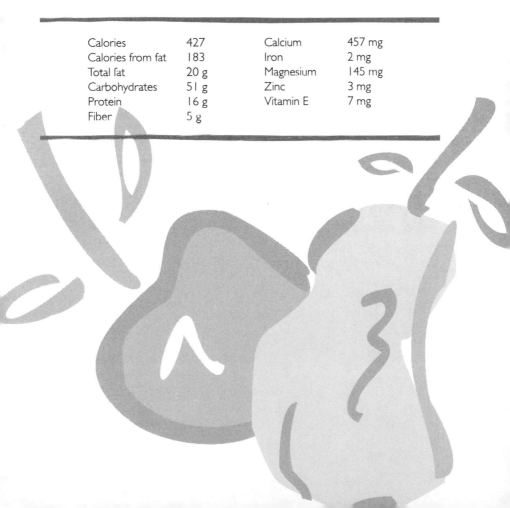

Peach Fling

This high-energy lunch drink will help to prevent afternoon let-down.

1 cup drained canned peaches

6 ounces lemon nonfat yogurt

1 to 2 tablespoons protein powder

1 teaspoon brewer's yeast

Calories	253	Riboflavin	0.4 mg
Calories from fat	9	Niacin	2 mg
Total fat	1 g	Thiamin	0.5 mg
Carbohydrates	47 g	Folic acid	122 mcg
Protein	18 g	Vitamin E	3 mg
Fiber	2 g		

Nutty Orange Shake

Here's a high-energy meal in a glass.

1 cup orange juice
1 cup milk of choice
1 frozen banana, cut into pieces
2 tablespoons almond butter
1 to 3 teaspoons MCT oil
1 tablespoon wheat germ

Calories	569	Iron	2 mg
Calories from fat	225	Magnesium	198 mg
Total fat	25 g	Thiamin	1 mg
Carbohydrates	76 g	Vitamin B6	1 mg
Protein	18 g	Folic acid	185 mcg
Fiber	6 g	Vitamin E	8 mg

Screaming Strawberry

For a garnish, add a small scoop of lime sorbet to the top of this smoothie.

1 cup frozen strawberries

1 cup strawberry nonfat yogurt

1 teaspoon brewer's yeast

1 tablespoon soy protein powder

1 teaspoon flaxseed oil

Calories	351	Calcium	367 mg
Calories from fat	72	Zinc	2 mg
Total fat	8 g	Riboflavin	1 mg
Carbohydrates	54 g	Folic acid	149 mcg
Protein	20 g	Vitamin E	2 mcg
Fiber	4 g		

Java Jolt

This smoothie is a cool, thick morning drink.

2 cups nonfat milk

1/2 cup frozen vanilla nonfat yogurt

1/2 frozen banana, cut into pieces

2 tablespoons instant coffee powder

2 tablespoons vanilla protein powder

1 teaspoon MCT oil

1 teaspoon brewer's yeast

1 teaspoon pure vanilla extract

Calories	468	Calcium	911 mg
Calories from fat	56	Magnesium	133 mg
Total fat	6 g	Potassium	1767 mg
Carbohydrates	59 g	Zinc	3 mg
Protein	43 g	Thiamin	1 mg
Fiber	1 g	Folic acid	154 mcg

Creamy Mint Tea

This recipe is for tired muscles. The magnesium and ginseng energize the muscles, while the caffeine in the tea reduces pain.

1 1/2 cups brewed green or black tea, cooled

3/4 cup vanilla lowfat frozen yogurt

4 to 6 fresh mint leaves

Powdered magnesium supplement (see label for recommended dosage)

Liquid ginseng supplement (see label for recommended dosage)

Calories	187	Iron	1 mg
Calories from fat	14	Magnesium	37 mg
Total fat	2 g	Potassium	395 mg
Carbohydrates	36 g	Zinc	1 mg
Protein	5 g	Riboflavin	0.3 mg
Fiber	0 g		

4

Power Makers
Smoothies for Athletes

A thletes make extraordinary demands of their bodies and therefore have special nutritional concerns. If you are a serious athlete, you should see a nutritionist or dietitian to develop a personal eating plan based on your individual physiology, the sport in which you compete, and your personal goals. The guidelines presented in this chapter will not apply to every person or every athletic endeavor, and the smoothie recipes are designed for training periods rather than for competitive events. See your coach, trainer, or nutritionist for more nutritional information.

GENERAL DIETARY RECOMMENDATIONS

Avoid salt. Too much salt can cause water retention and weight gain.

Keep hydrated during exercise. Water is necessary to regulate body temperature and is especially important for athletes involved in endurance-type exercise. Even modest exercise requires a quart of water for every 1,000 calories ingested.

Avoid caffeine. Caffeine is often a potent diuretic, which can cause dehydration.

Avoid a diet that is high in fat and high in animal protein. More protein does not translate into larger muscles.

SMOOTHIE INGREDIENTS FOR ATHLETES AND BODY BUILDERS

Avocados

Avocados are an excellent source of potassium and vitamin E as well as the heart-healthy monounsaturated fatty acids. Avocado slices blend easily into smoothies, where they increase the caloric content.

Brewer's Yeast

As the intake of calories rise, the need for the B vitamins also increases. This powder is an inexpensive way to supplement the diet with the B vitamins necessary for carbohydrate metabolism. It mixes easily with liquids.

Creatine

Creatine supplements may be of benefit to those involved in sprinting-type events, such as running or swimming, or exercise of intermittent intensity or team sports, such as football, basketball, or tennis. In a study published in the *Journal of the American Dietetic Association*, seven weight lifters who took twenty-five grams of creatine monohydrate daily for a week were able to lift more weight and also gained an average of one to two pounds more than seven weight trainers given placebo. Creatine absorption by muscle tissue is enhanced by insulin, so it should be taken with meals or fruit juice or drink with a high glycemic index (a food that stimulates insulin production).

Iron

Athletes involved in marathon-type sports such as running, military march, and endurance bicycle riding can develop low iron levels as the result of a slow blood loss through intestinal bleeding. Some protein powders contain supplemental iron. Iron is also contained in sea vegetables, such as spirulina, dulse, and algae, and in dates, prunes, and prune juice. Vitamin C added to an iron-containing smoothie will enhance the absorption of iron.

Magnesium

Endurance exercise changes the concentration of magnesium in muscle tissue and blood. As levels of hormones such as adrenaline increase, there is an increase in the urinary loss of magnesium. This mineral may improve muscle strength in athletes. Magnesium is available as a liquid in health food stores. Or you can use bananas, blueberries, carrot juice, cherries, dates, grapefruit, oranges, tomato juice, and raspberries to add magnesium to your smoothies.

Potassium

Exercise causes a loss of potassium, a trace mineral essential for proper muscle function. Without sufficient potassium, muscles easily become fatigued. All fruits are sources of potassium.

Protein Powders

Protein powders are available in a wide variety of flavors with a wide variety of additives designed especially for athletes and body builders. Look for a protein mix that contains a creatine supplement. Protein powders made from soy also bring the benefits of soy isoflavones.

Pyridoxine

Exercisers and athletes often have low pyridoxine (vitamin B6) levels. Exercise causes vitamin B6 blood levels to increase because of the release of enzymes from muscle that require the presence of this vitamin. This leaves less B6 available for other needs of the body.

Seeds and Nuts

Rich in natural heart-healthy oils, seeds and nuts also contain fat-soluble vitamins, essential fatty acids, and minerals, such as calcium and zinc. There is an increased need for all of these nutrients in muscle building. Add ground nuts and seeds, including tahini (ground sesame seeds), sunflower seed butter, almond butter, peanut butter, and cashew butter, to smoothies.

Soy Milk

Full-fat (whole), fortified soy milk contains no saturated fat or cholesterol and is a healthy source of protein and polyunsaturated fat for all athletes of all levels. Soy milk also contains a multitude of protective phytonutrients, which aid in the prevention of cancer, heart disease, and osteoporosis, a disease that often affects women athletes.

Tofu

This soy food contains all of the benefits of tofu plus those of fiber. Soft or silken tofu is a rich source of essential fatty acids, protein, calcium, and magnesium and can be incorporated into any smoothie recipe.

La Playa Power

This is a calorie-rich and protein-rich drink for the serious athlete.

1 cup lowfat coconut milk

1 cup pineapple pieces, canned or fresh, juice included

1 frozen banana, cut into pieces

3 tablespoons protein powder

1 tablespoon flaxseed powder

1 teaspoon flaxseed oil

Calories	663	Iron	10 mg
Calories from fat	251	Magnesium	242 mg
Total fat	28 g	Potassium	1667 mg
Carbohydrates	87 g	Zinc	9 mg
Protein	18 g	Niacin	15 mg
Fiber	6 g	Vitamin E	10 mg

Tropical Elixir

The pineapple in this drink acts to reduce inflammation in the muscles caused by exercise.

1 cup fresh pineapple pieces

1 cup vanilla nonfat yogurt

1/2 cup lowfat coconut milk

3 tablespoons protein powder

1 tablespoon brewer's yeast

Calories	553	Calcium	771 mg
Calories from fat	101	Iron	6 mg
Total fat	11 g	Magnesium	180 mg
Carbohydrates	84 g	Zinc	110 mg
Protein	30 g	Niacin	17 mg
Fiber	2 g	Vitamin E	8 mg

The Pump

Tahini (ground sesame seeds) adds flavor, calories, and healthy oils to this drink.

1 cup nonfat milk

1 cup strawberries

1 frozen banana, cut into pieces

2 tablespoons protein powder

2 tablespoons tahini (ground sesame seeds)

1 tablespoon flaxseed oil

1 tablespoon lecithin granules

Liquid calcium/magnesium supplement (see label for recommended dosage)

2 to 3 grams creatine powder (see label for recommended dosage)

Calories	740	Iron	5 mg
Calories from fat	404	Potassium	1568 mg
Total fat	45 g	Zinc	8 mg
Carbohydrates	72 g	Vitamin A	250 mcg
Protein	24 g	Vitamin E	13 mg
Fiber	9 g		

Chocolate Peanut Butter Heaven

The peanut butter and flaxseed are sources of heart-healthy fat, calories, and fiber.

1 cup whole soy milk

1 cup vanilla nonfat frozen yogurt

2 tablespoons chocolate sauce or cocoa powder

2 tablespoons vanilla protein powder

2 tablespoons flaxseed powder

2 tablespoons natural-style peanut butter

Calories	776	Iron	11 mg
Calories from fat	247	Zinc	8 mg
Total fat	27 g	Niacin	13 mg
Carbohydrates	99 g	Thiamin	1 mg
Protein	37 g	Vitamin E	8 mg
Fiber	7 g		

The Works Shake

The name says it all! This drink provides everything an athlete needs to build and maintain lean tissue mass.

1 cup whole soy milk

1 frozen banana, cut into pieces

1/2 cup orange juice concentrate

3 tablespoons protein powder

1 tablespoon flaxseed oil

1 tablespoon lecithin granules

1 tablespoon brewer's yeast

500 mg calcium as a liquid

1 to 3 grams creatine powder (see label for
    recommended dosage)

Calories	807	Iron	5 mg
Calories from fat	294	Zinc	8 mg
Total fat	33 g	Folic acid	657 mcg
Carbohydrates	113 g	Vitamin C	219 mg
Protein	27 g	Vitamin E	15 mg
Calcium	828 mg		

Piña Colada

This is a smooth-tasting recovery drink. Fresh pineapple is a source of bromelain, which reduces inflammation, and potassium, an electrolyte lost during exercise.

1 1/2 cups fresh pineapple juice

1/3 cup lowfat coconut milk

1/2 cup frozen pineapple chunks

1 tablespoon lecithin granules

Calories	487	Iron	3 mg
Calories from fat	186	Magnesium	98 mg
Total fat	21 g	Potassium	787 mg
Carbohydrates	80 g	Vitamin B6	1 mg
Protein	2 g	Folic acid	110 mcg
Fiber	2 g		

Pete's Marathon

Raspberries are one of the richest sources of salicylates, nature's aspirin. They can help to reduce inflammation and pain following exercise. The banana replaces lost potassium, and the orange juice refuels the muscles with glucose.

1 cup frozen raspberries

1 cup rice milk

1/2 frozen banana, cut into pieces

2 tablespoons orange juice concentrate

Calories	223	Fiber	10 g
Calories from fat	12	Iron	1 mg
Total fat	1 g	Potassium	676 mg
Carbohydrates	54 g	Vitamin B6	1 mg
Protein	57 g	Folic acid	100 mcg

Eggnog

Here's a festive way to get your protein.

1 cup nonfat eggnog

1/2 cup nonfat milk

3 tablespoons protein powder

1 tablespoon flaxseed powder

1 teaspoon fresh ground nutmeg

1 teaspoon brewer's yeast

Calories	353	Calcium	582 mg
Calories from fat	34	Iron	5 mg
Total fat	4 g	Zinc	8 mg
Carbohydrates	56 g	Vitamin A	500 mcg
Protein	23 g	Vitamin E	8 mg
Fiber	1 g		

Iron Pump

This drink is rich in iron, to replace losses caused by intestinal bleeding from prolonged exercise. The vitamin C from the orange juice helps the body to absorb the iron.

1 orange, peeled and seeded

1 frozen banana, cut into pieces

4 soaked prunes

1 tablespoon blackstrap molasses

1 teaspoon algae

Calories	303	Fiber	9 g
Calories from fat	10	Iron	6 mg
Total fat	1 g	Magnesium	110 mg
Carbohydrates	76 g	Potassium	1477 mg
Protein	5 g	Vitamin B6	1 mg

Super Hero

This smoothie is a great base for supplements. The frozen strawberries hide the often gritty texture of some protein products, and the lecithin keeps oils emulsified.

1 cup whole soy milk

1/2 cup orange juice concentrate

1 cup frozen strawberries

1 tablespoon lecithin granules

Calories	455	Iron	2 mg
Calories from fat	171	Magnesium	110 mg
Total fat	19 g	Thiamin	1 mg
Carbohydrates	69 g	Folic acid	252 mcg
Protein	11 g	Vitamin C	281 mg
Fiber	8 g		

Dated Mango

The dates add sweetness as well as trace minerals to this smoothie.

1 cup whole soy milk

1 cup frozen mango slices

1/2 cup vanilla nonfat yogurt

1/2 cup chopped dates

2 tablespoons protein powder

1 tablespoon lecithin granules

1 tablespoon flaxseed oil

Calories	854	Magnesium	155 mg
Calories from fat	296	Zinc	7 mg
Total fat	33 g	Vitamin B6	1 mg
Carbohydrates	132 g	Beta carotene	1113 mcg
Protein	24 g	Vitamin E	14 mg
Fiber	10 g		

Honey and Nut Pounder

The sweet flavors of honey and nuts combine to make this smoothie a real winner.

1 cup whole soy milk

1 cup vanilla nonfat yogurt

1 banana

2 tablespoons vanilla protein powder

3 tablespoons almond butter

1 tablespoon honey

1 teaspoon pure almond extract

Calories	751	Calcium	726 mg
Calories from fat	221	Iron	4 mg
Total fat	25 g	Magnesium	262 mg
Carbohydrates	105 g	Zinc	9 mg
Protein	34 g	Niacin	11 mg
Fiber	7 g	Vitamin E	12 mg

Nutty Tropical Blonde

The coconut milk and almond butter add a rich, smooth taste to this smoothie.

1 cup lowfat coconut milk

1/2 cup pineapple chunks

1/2 cup mango slices

1/2 cup guava nectar

1 banana

2 tablespoons almond butter

2 tablespoons protein powder

Calories	811	Iron	7 mg
Calories from fat	358	Magnesium	298 mg
Total fat	40 g	Zinc	8 mg
Carbohydrates	102 g	Vitamin A	450 mcg
Protein	17 g	Vitamin E	13 mg
Fiber	7 g		

CHAPTER 5

Calorie Burners

Smoothies for Weight Loss

*T*he "secret" to weight loss is simple: Take in fewer calories than you burn. The difficulty lies in keeping the weight off. Appetite and energy regulation are extremely complicated and poorly understood processes, involving a complex interplay between neurotransmitters, genetics, food choices, and exercise. This chapter offers meal replacement drinks made with whole foods. They can help you avoid the quick, yet often fatty foods eaten by busy people on the run. By themselves they will not cause you to lose weight. However, if you substitute them for high calorie refined food fatty meals, these drinks will help you to keep your appetite under control while providing your body with needed nutrients.

The meal replacement smoothies in this chapter are cheaper and superior to the canned variety. Stored properly, most of the ingredients are not perishable and can easily be kept on hand. When designing your smoothie meal replacements, include some fat in your smoothie recipes. This is most easily done with full-fat or lowfat soy milk. The butterfat found in milk and yogurt is high in saturated fat, whereas the fat in soy milk, nuts, and seeds is heart-healthy vegetable fat.

Diets that are high in carbohydrates and low in protein may help to increase brain levels of the neurotransmitter serotonin, which improves mood and decreases appetite. In a study of forty obese women with a history of diet failure due to stress-related overeating, MIT researcher Judith Wurtman found that those who consumed a 1,400-calorie, high-carbohydrate, low-protein diet had fewer cravings and better overall moods and lost more weight than those who followed a high-protein, low-carbohydrate diet of the same calories.

GENERAL DIETARY RECOMMENDATIONS

Set realistic goals. You do not have to diet down to your so-called "ideal" weight to reap the rewards of weight loss. A ten-pound loss can make a big difference to your health: it can lower blood pressure, decrease cholesterol levels, and improve glucose tolerance.

Balance each meal so that it contains some fat, fiber, and protein. Fat, fiber, and protein all increase the amount of time food spends in the stomach. This allows the carbohydrates in the meal to enter your bloodstream slowly so that insulin (which promotes fat storage) levels do not sharply rise. This steady stream of glucose also keeps you from getting hungry again too soon.

Eat five or six small meals instead of three large ones. Large meals promote fat storage. Smaller, more frequent meals keep glucose levels more even.

Always eat breakfast. Your brain and muscles need food to replenish stores after the overnight fast, and its calories are more likely to be burned for energy.

Eat your largest meal before six in the evening. Calories eaten in the evening tend to be stored as fat rather than burned for energy.

Avoid refined foods. This means foods made with white sugar and white flour.

Take a chromium supplement to improve the way your body regulates insulin.

SMOOTHIE INGREDIENTS TO PROMOTE WEIGHT LOSS

Brewer's Yeast

This powder is an inexpensive way to supplement the diet with the B vitamins necessary for carbohydrate metabolism. It is mild tasting, which makes it the ideal smoothie supplement. Brewer's yeast is an excellent source of the chromium-containing glucose tolerance factor. This complex regulates insulin and glucose tolerance, decreasing appetite and promoting weight loss.

Caffeine

Caffeine is a natural plant alkaloid that may stimulate the metabolism and fat loss. One teaspoon of instant coffee powder will add 65 mg of caffeine to your smoothie, and one teaspoon of instant tea powder will add 30 mg. Five ounces of brewed tea will add 40 mg.

Carbohydrates

Carbohydrates enhance the uptake of the amino acid tryptophan by the brain, where it is converted into serotonin, the neurotransmitter responsible for mood. Some people will find that a high-carbohydrate drink will decrease their appetite, relieve stress, and help them to lose weight. All fruits are excellent sources of nutrient-rich carbohydrates.

Conjugated Linolenic Acid

Conjugated linolenic acid, or CLA, is a naturally occurring fat that may enhance the loss of fat while increasing the gain of muscle. Animal studies at University of Wisconsin at Madison show CLA significantly reduces fat and appetite while increasing muscle. Human studies are now under way. CLA supplements can be purchased at health food stores and are often used by bodybuilders and other athletes.

Fiber

All whole foods are good sources of fiber, which is necessary for elimination and intestinal function. Prunes, dates, psyllium seed powder, flaxseed powder, and oat and wheat bran are particularly fiber-rich. Because fiber is often neglected on a low-calorie diet, add one of these high-fiber ingredients to your smoothie when you are dieting. Fiber will also increase the time the smoothie spends in your stomach so that blood sugar levels rise evenly and keep you satiated.

Ginger

Ginger is an herb that may be able to increase the metabolism. Add ginger root powder to smoothies or crush a piece of peeled fresh ginger root.

Protein Powders

Add soy or milk protein to balance out the carbohydrate content of the smoothie. Protein is needed to burn fat properly. High insulin levels promote fat storage, and protein powders can help to keep the body's insulin levels even.

Sea Vegetables

Kelp, dulse, algae, spirulina, and other sea vegetables are rich in chromium. Chromium allows glucose to enter cells and is a vital trace mineral in the metabolism of fat, sugars, and proteins. Sea vegetables are also sources of iron, a mineral in which many women are deficient.

Stevia

Stevia is a natural plant extract. It contains no carbohydrates and is naturally sweet. Some researchers believe stevia has the potential for inhibiting fat absorption and decreasing hypertension. Stevia is available in liquid or powdered form. Use it in any smoothie to increase sweetness.

Wheat Germ

Wheat germ is a source of fiber necessary for regularity when dieting. Each tablespoon of wheat germ adds one gram of protein, two grams of fiber, vitamin E, and a variety of phytochemicals.

Berry Morning

This is the best way to start the day! Always keep a variety of frozen fruit in the freezer so it is available when you get hungry.

1/2 cup fortified milk of choice

1/2 cup frozen or fresh berries of choice (such as strawberries, blackberries, raspberries)

1/2 fresh banana

2 tablespoons protein powder

1 tablespoon wheat germ

1 teaspoon brewer's yeast

Calories	219	Calcium	227 mg
Calories from fat	19	Iron	1 mg
Total fat	2 g	Zinc	2 mg
Carbohydrates	29 g	Thiamin	1 mg
Protein	25 g	Vitamin B6	1 mg
Fiber	4 g	Folic acid	154 mcg

Banana Light

Thick and smooth, with a delicate flavor, this smoothie will fill you up without filling you out.

1 cup rice milk

1 frozen banana, cut into pieces

1/2 cup ice

1 teaspoon pure vanilla extract

Calories	169	Fiber	3 g
Calories from fat	7	Magnesium	42 mg
Total fat	1 g	Potassium	478 mg
Carbohydrates	40 g	Vitamin B6	1 mg
Protein	55 g		

Breakfast Smoothie

Buy soy milk in aseptic containers so that it is readily available.

10 ounces cocoa fortified whole soy milk

1 banana (fresh or frozen), cut into pieces

2 tablespoons cocoa protein powder

1 tablespoon brewer's yeast

1 tablespoon wheat germ

1/2 teaspoon ground cinnamon

Calories	415	Iron	5 mg
Calories from fat	61	Magnesium	106 mg
Total fat	7 g	Zinc	2 mg
Carbohydrates	62 g	Niacin	5 mg
Protein	32 g	Thiamin	2 mg
Fiber	10 g	Folic acid	403 mcg

Energy Shake

Chewable CLA supplement can be crushed and added to smoothies.

1 1/2 cups milk of choice

1 frozen banana, cut into pieces

3 tablespoons cocoa powder

Pyruvate and conjugated linolenic acid powdered supplement (see label for recommended dosage)

1 to 3 grams creatine powder (see label for recommended dosage)

Liquid magnesium supplement (see label for recommended dosage)

Calories	297	Calcium	478 mg
Calories from fat	30	Iron	3 mg
Total fat	3 g	Magnesium	150 mg
Carbohydrates	53 g	Potassium	1288 mg
Protein	17 g	Zinc	3 mg
Fiber	3 g	Vitamin A	234 mcg

Morning Glory

Psyllium seed powder is an excellent source of soluble fiber. Soluble fiber feeds the healthy bacteria in your colon, promoting regularity and reducing cholesterol.

1 cup frozen strawberries

1/2 cup plain nonfat yogurt

1/2 banana

1 tablespoon brewer's yeast

1 teaspoon psyllium seed powder

Calories	186	Calcium	267 mg
Calories from fat	10	Iron	2 mg
Total fat	1 g	Niacin	4 mg
Carbohydrates	39 g	Thiamin	1 mg
Protein	11 g	Vitamin B6	1 mg
Fiber	8 g	Folic acid	364 mcg

Afternoon Chocolate De-Lite

For those weekends when you must have a chocolate shake. This thick and creamy alternative is low in fat and rich in protein and complex carbohydrates. It is also the perfect way to introduce tofu to children.

1 cup fresh or frozen raspberries

1/2 cup nonfat milk

1/2 cup well-chilled silken tofu

3 tablespoons cocoa powder

1 teaspoon flaxseed powder

Calories	274	Fiber	9 g
Calories from fat	81	Calcium	370 mg
Total fat	9 g	Iron	6 mg
Carbohydrates	32 g	Magnesium	117 mg
Protein	18 g	Zinc	2 mg

Peachy Almond Freeze

Thick and rich, this fiber-rich smoothie has a delicate almond flavor. For a thicker smoothie, use frozen peaches.

1 cup almond milk

1/2 cup frozen or drained canned peaches

1 teaspoon spirulina

1 teaspoon psyllium seed powder

1 to 2 drops pure almond extract

Calories	317	Iron	3 mg
Calories from fat	221	Magnesium	154 mg
Total fat	25 g	Zinc	2 mg
Carbohydrates	17 g	Riboflavin	1 mg
Protein	13 g	Niacin	3 mg
Fiber	5 g	Vitamin E	12 mg

Granola Shake

This is a great breakfast drink.

1 cup lowfat milk of choice
1/4 cup lowfat granola
1/2 cup vanilla nonfat yogurt
1 frozen banana, cut into pieces

Calories	406	Calcium	543 mg
Calories from fat	43	Magnesium	109 mg
Total fat	5 g	Zinc	4 mg
Carbohydrates	76 g	Niacin	3 mg
Protein	18 g	Vitamin E	5 mg
Fiber	4 g		

Chocolate Almond

Here's a light chocolate drink rich in protein—perfect for an afternoon pick-me-up.

1 cup almond milk

1/2 cup ice

2 tablespoons protein powder

1 tablespoon flaxseed powder

1 tablespoon chocolate syrup

Calories	449	Calcium	226 mg
Calories from fat	270	Iron	9 mg
Total fat	30 g	Magnesium	174 mg
Carbohydrates	19 g	Zinc	2 mg
Protein	30 g	Vitamin E	11 mg
Fiber	1 g		

Berry Froth

This smoothie is a good source of potassium. Many people feel better taking potassium during weight-loss programs.

1 cup fortified nonfat soy milk

1/2 cup frozen mixed berries

1/2 frozen banana, cut into pieces

2 tablespoons protein powder

1 teaspoon lecithin granules

1 teaspoon brewer's yeast

Calories	255	Calcium	273 mg
Calories from fat	51	Iron	2 mg
Total fat	6 g	Thiamin	1 mg
Carbohydrates	34 g	Vitamin B6	0.4 mg
Protein	23 g	Folic acid	127 mcg
Fiber	3 g		

Melon Slush

Melon provides fiber and flavor with a minimum of calories. For a sweeter drink, add stevia, a natural noncarbohydrate sweetener.

1 cup frozen cantaloupe and honeydew pieces

1/2 cup orange juice

1/2 cup filtered water

Stevia to taste, optional

Calories	112	Potassium	733 mg
Calories from fat	5	Niacin	1 mg
Total fat	1 g	Folic acid	82 mcg
Carbohydrates	27 g	Vitamin C	64 mg
Protein	2 g	Beta carotene	4810 mcg
Fiber	1 g		

Iced Tropical Blonde

The coconut extract adds a hint of coconut flavor without the calories.

1/4 cup fresh pineapple chunks

1/4 cup mango slices

1 frozen banana, cut into pieces

1/2 teaspoon coconut extract

Calories	159	Magnesium	42 mg
Calories from fat	7	Potassium	566 mg
Total fat	1 g	Vitamin B6	1 mg
Carbohydrates	39 g	Folic acid	32 mcg
Protein	2 g	Vitamin A	171 mcg
Fiber	4 g		

Peaches and Cottage Cheese

Enjoy this smoothie as a lunchtime meal replacement.

1 cup drained canned peaches

1 cup nonfat cottage cheese

1 tablespoon wheat germ

Calories	261	Calcium	174 mg
Calories from fat	7	Magnesium	30 mg
Total fat	1 g	Zinc	1 mg
Carbohydrates	29 g	Vitamin A	144 mcg
Protein	33 g	Vitamin E	4 mg
Fiber	3 g		

CHAPTER 6

Immunizers

Smoothies to Build the Immune System

our immune system is like an army. Its soldiers patrol the high-ways and byways of your blood stream and tissues, on a search-and-destroy mission for bacterial, viral, and fungal invaders. A poor diet produces weak soldiers and builds ineffective weapons, leaving the body open to colds, flu, pneumonia, and even cancer. Smoothies offer the op-portunity to add nutrients and herbs to your diet that you might other-wise miss.

Immune-building smoothies can aid in the prevention and recov-ery from illness. They can help to support your body until you feel like eating solid food again, and they are often attractive when solid food is not appetizing.

GENERAL DIETARY RECOMMENDATIONS

Limit the amount of alcohol you drink. Alcohol can deplete the im-mune system of nutrients.

Eat generous amounts of garlic and onions. The sulfur-containing compounds in these foods stimulate the immune system.

Eat foods high in copper and zinc. These trace minerals are necessary for a proper-functioning immune system. Nuts, whole grains, and legumes are good sources of all the trace minerals.

SMOOTHIE INGREDIENTS TO BUILD THE IMMUNE SYSTEM

Acidophilus

Acidophilus milk or 1/2 teaspoon of acidophilus powder or liquid supplement can be added to help replenish the healthy bacteria in the colon that are killed during antibiotic treatments. These bacteria can also be found in yogurt.

Algae

Algae is valuable to the immune system because of its trace mineral content. An iron deficiency reduces the ability of natural killer cells to destroy cancerous cells and engulf bacteria and viruses and decreases the ability of neutrophils to kill. Algae such as chlorella or spirulina are also sources of the antioxidant chlorophyll. Add one teaspoon to smoothies.

L-Arginine

Arginine is an amino acid that, apart from its role in protein synthesis, can act as an immune system enhancer. Researchers have found that arginine can stimulate the thymus gland and increase the production of the white blood cells, which attack bacteria and viruses. Arginine can be purchased in a powdered form. Add 300 to 400 mg of arginine to a smoothie.

Brewer's Yeast

This supplement is an excellent source of the B complex vitamins, including B6. Vitamin B6, or pyridoxine, is necessary for the formation of antibodies. A B6 deficiency results in a decrease in lymphocytes (a type of white blood cell) and reduces lymphocytes response to chemical messages for help from T and B lymphocytes.

Chlorophyll

Chlorophyll is the magnesium-containing green pigment found in plants that is responsible for photosynthesis. In the human body, chlorophyll can act as an antioxidant, neutralizing free radicals and protecting against cancer and environmental toxins. Wheat grass and other fresh green vegetable juices are sources of chlorophyll. Or you can add one teaspoon of liquid or powdered extract to a smoothie.

Orange-Colored Fruits and Vegetables

These fruits and vegetables are rich in the antioxidant beta carotene. beta carotene protects the cells from being injured by free radicals generated by the immune system. They are also a source of vitamin A, which improves antibody response and increases the production of certain white blood cells (natural killer cells, macrophages, T cells). Good smoothie additions are papayas, mangoes, peaches, apricots, pink grapefruits, and carrot juice.

Propolis

Propolis is a resin that bees collect from the buds of trees and flowers. It contains a natural antibiotic called galangin, which is purported to prevent low-grade infections and stimulate the immune system. Propolis is said to enhance the effectiveness of conventional antibiotics such as penicillin and streptomycin.

Protein

Most people get more than enough protein from their diets; however, dieters, children, vegans, and those who are ill may not be getting enough protein to keep their immune army in shape. Add a scoop of any protein powder to boost the immune-building properties of your smoothie. Plain yogurt, soy milk, tofu, and dairy milk will also add protein to your smoothies.

Vitamin C

Vitamin C (ascorbic acid) is a powerful antioxidant that protects the watery areas of the cell from free radical damage; it also helps to protect the white blood cells from the oxidizing agents produced by neutrophils, a type of white blood cell. Vitamin C also enhances the effect of antibiotic therapy and detoxifies histamine, a substance that can suppress the immune system. Only 500 mg of vitamin C is needed to saturate tissues to prevent respiratory infections, and therapeutic doses of one to four grams have been shown to reduce the duration of a cold by almost half. Ascorbic acid is available in powdered form. Vitamin C–rich foods, such as cherries, lemons, limes, oranges, papayas, strawberries, tangerines, and grapefruits, can also be added to smoothies to help strengthen the immune system. These foods also contain flavonoids and other immune-boosting substances.

Wheat Germ

Wheat germ is the nutrient-dense part of the wheat berry. It contains vitamin E, some B vitamins, magnesium, and zinc. Only one tablespoon of wheat germ will add 2 grams of protein and 1 gram of fiber to your smoothie.

Yogurt

Yogurt is milk that is treated with strains of friendly bacteria, such as *Lactobacillus bulgaricus, Lactobacillus acidophilus,* and *Streptococcus thermophilus.* These bacteria promote the regrowth of the healthy microflora in the gut after they have been killed by antibiotics. Be sure to purchase yogurt with live cultures (this will be marked on the label). Frozen yogurt does not contain live cultures, so always use fresh. Yogurt also contains an unidentified antibiotic factor that helps prevent infection in women, and it makes yogurt a valuable food for those with immune problems.

Zinc

The mineral zinc is involved with almost ninety enzyme systems in the body. A deficiency in this mineral leads to a decrease in the number of T cells and natural killer cells, leaving cells vulnerable to infection. Zinc supplementation is shown to increase the number of white blood cells and inhibit the growth of bacteria. Zinc is often added to protein powders.

HERBS TO BUILD THE IMMUNE SYSTEM

Echinacea

The root of *Echinacea purpurea,* commonly called echinacea, contains substances called arabinogalactans, which stimulate the immune response to protect the body from viruses and bacteria. This herb also reduces the side effects associated with chemotherapy, making it especially suited for those with cancer.

Ginseng

Chinese or Korean ginseng (*Panax ginseng*) has been used by Asian cultures for centuries as a tonic, stimulant, and rejuvenator. Ginseng's healing properties are believed due to a family of poorly understood chemicals called ginsenosides. Ginseng stimulates the cells of the reticuloendothelial system, the part of the immune system that contains macrophages, the white blood cells that eat bacteria and viral particles. It also enhances antibody response and the production of interferon. You can add ginseng extract or liquid to smoothies.

Goldenseal

This native American herb contains an alkaloid called berberine, which has demonstrated antibiotic and immune system stimulatory properties. Berberine inhibits the growth of candida, a type of yeast that often causes infections after antibiotic usage. Goldenseal extracts can be purchased at health food stores.

Licorice

Licorice root extract is a natural immune stimulant. Its main active ingredient is glycyrrhizin, which can act as an antioxidant that preserves vitamin E, protects the heart, and supports anticancer activity. It also contains isoflavones, which are thought to prevent hormone-related cancers. In the test tube, licorice shows antibacterial action.

Tea

The powerful antioxidant polyphenols found in tea (catechins found in green tea and theaflavins and thearubigens found in black tea) may confer antiviral, antibacterial, and antifungal properties. They help prevent the development of cancer, inhibit the multiplication of viruses, guard against food-borne pathogenic bacteria, and protect teeth from cavity-inducing bacteria.

Pauling's Punch

This smoothie is rich in vitamin C and the bioflavonoids.

1/2 cup orange juice

1/2 cup plain nonfat yogurt

1/2 lemon, peeled and seeded

1/2 grapefruit, peeled and seeded

1/2 cup ice

1 (1-inch) piece fresh ginger root, peeled
and crushed

1 tablespoon molasses

Calories	220	Calcium	281 mg
Calories from fat	6	Magnesium	77 mg
Total fat	1 g	Potassium	866 mg
Carbohydrates	46 g	Folic acid	80 mcg
Protein	9 g	Vitamin C	88 mg
Fiber	2 g		

Papaya Tea

Fresh papaya contains the anti-inflammatory enzyme papain. This antioxidant-rich smoothie is easy on an irritated stomach.

8 ounces brewed green or black tea, cooled

1/2 cup papaya slices

3 to 4 ice cubes

200 to 300 mg vitamin C powder

Calories	30	Fiber	1 g
Calories from fat	1	Potassium	268 mg
Total fat	0 g	Vitamin C	243 mg
Carbohydrates	7 g	Vitamin A	141 mcg
Protein	0 g		

Antioxidant Elixir

Fresh pineapple contains the immune-enhancing enzyme bromelain.

1 cup orange juice

1/2 apple, cored, peeled, and sliced

1/2 cup fresh or frozen pineapple chunks

1/2 cup ice

1 teaspoon algae

Calories	205	Iron	2 mg
Calories from fat	10	Magnesium	48 mg
Total fat	1 g	Thiamin	0.4 mg
Carbohydrates	48 g	Folic acid	119 mcg
Protein	5 g	Vitamin C	113 mg
Fiber	3 g	Vitamin A	139 mcg

Strawberry Smoothie

This smoothie is great for sore throats. It can be used as a meal replacement when whole soy milk is used.

1/2 cup nonfat milk or any soy milk

1/2 cup frozen strawberries

1/2 cup vanilla lowfat frozen yogurt

1 tablespoon honey

Calories	251	Calcium	223 mg
Calories from fat	14	Iron	1 mg
Total fat	2 g	Potassium	498 mg
Carbohydrates	51 g	Riboflavin	0.4 mg
Protein	8 g	Vitamin C	43 mg
Fiber	2 g		

Rasanana Berry

All berries are rich in antiviral and antibiotic compounds as well as the immune-enhancing vitamin C.

1/2 cup almond milk

1/2 frozen banana, cut into pieces

1/2 cup strawberries

1/4 cup raspberries

1/4 cup blueberries

1 tablespoon brewer's yeast

Calories	268	Fiber	6 g
Calories from fat	117	Iron	3 mg
Total fat	13 g	Magnesium	101 mg
Carbohydrates	32 g	Folic acid	361 mcg
Protein	9 g	Vitamin E	6 mg

Watermelon Antioxidant

The flavorings in the echinacea extract will not clash with the light flavor of the watermelon. Watermelon is a source of lycopene, a powerful antioxidant from the carotene family.

1 1/2 cups watermelon pieces, seedless

1/2 cup ice

500 mg vitamin C powder

Echinacea extract (see label for
   recommended dosage)

Calories	76	Potassium	281 mg
Calories from fat	9	Vitamin B6	0.3 mg
Total fat	1 g	Vitamin C	523 mg
Carbohydrates	17 g	Vitamin A	88 mcg
Protein	2 g	Beta carotene	555 mcg
Fiber	1 g		

Orange Cooler

This is an unusual blend of carrots and apricots and is rich in the immune-stimulating carotenes.

1 cup fresh carrot juice

1 cup drained canned apricots

1/2 cup orange juice

300 to 400 mg L-arginine powder

Calories	234	Iron	2 mg
Calories from fat	5	Potassium	1235 mg
Total fat	1 g	Folic acid	67 mcg
Carbohydrates	57 g	Vitamin C	78 mg
Protein	4 g	Vitamin A	6628 mcg
Fiber	5 g	Beta carotene	25846 mcg

Honeyed Apple with a Secret

This smoothie contains a secret ingredient: garlic. Apples contain an antiviral compound that make this drink a good choice for preventing winter infections.

1 cup apple juice

1 apple, cored, peeled, and sliced

1/2 cup orange juice

1 (2-inch) piece fresh ginger root, peeled and chopped

1 clove garlic, peeled and chopped

1 tablespoon honey

500 mg vitamin C powder

Echinacea extract, optional (see label for recommended dosage)

Calories	375	Iron	2 mg
Calories from fat	13	Magnesium	61 mg
Total fat	1 g	Potassium	1048 mg
Carbohydrates	91 g	Folic acid	56 mcg
Protein	3 g	Vitamin C	561 mg
Fiber	4 g		

Cherry Buzz

This smoothie combines propolis and honey, two products of bees that have immune-enhancing properties.

1 cup frozen cherries, pitted

1/2 cup orange juice

1/2 lemon, peeled and seeded

1 tablespoon honey

1 tablespoon propolis

Calories	234	Magnesium	32 mg
Calories from fat	14	Potassium	613 mg
Total fat	2 g	Niacin	1 mg
Carbohydrates	57 g	Folic acid	65 mcg
Protein	3 g	Vitamin C	74 mg
Fiber	4 g		

Snappy Mango Shake

Fresh ginger root adds a snap to this thick mango shake.

1 cup mango pieces

1/2 cup nonfat acidophilus milk

1/2 fresh banana

1 (2-inch) piece fresh ginger root, peeled and crushed

200 to 300 mg vitamin C powder

Calories	266	Niacin	2 mg
Calories from fat	14	Vitamin B6	1 mg
Total fat	2 g	Vitamin C	258 mg
Carbohydrates	60 g	Vitamin A	740 mcg
Protein	7 g	Beta carotene	528 mcg
Fiber	5 g	Vitamin E	2 mg

Blueberry Shake

This drink makes a good base for flavored herbs because blueberries have a mild sweet flavor that blends well with the strong flavoring of herbal supplements.

1 cup frozen blueberries

1 cup milk of choice

1 fresh banana

Liquid herbal supplement (see label for
   recommended dosage)

Calories	272	Fiber	7 g
Calories from fat	14	Calcium	318 mg
Total fat	2 g	Potassium	986 mg
Carbohydrates	59 g	Riboflavin	1 mg
Protein	11 g	Vitamin B6	1 mg

Cocoa Coconut

This recipe has two of Danni's favorite flavors! This drink teams the smoothness of coconut with the antiviral properties of raspberries and the immune-enhancing properties of cocoa's resveratrol.

1 1/2 cups frozen raspberries

1/2 cup lowfat coconut milk

1 banana

1/4 cup cocoa powder

2 tablespoons shredded coconut

2 tablespoons cocoa soy protein powder

1 tablespoon brewer's yeast

Calories	550	Iron	8 mg
Calories from fat	198	Magnesium	231 mg
Total fat	22 g	Zinc	3 mg
Carbohydrates	66 g	Folic acid	408 mcg
Protein	29 g	Vitamin C	57 mg
Fiber	17 g		

Creamed Apricots

This drink teams the antibiotic properties of yogurt with the antioxidant properties of beta carotene.

1 cup canned apricots with juice

1 cup plain nonfat yogurt

1/2 cup pineapple juice

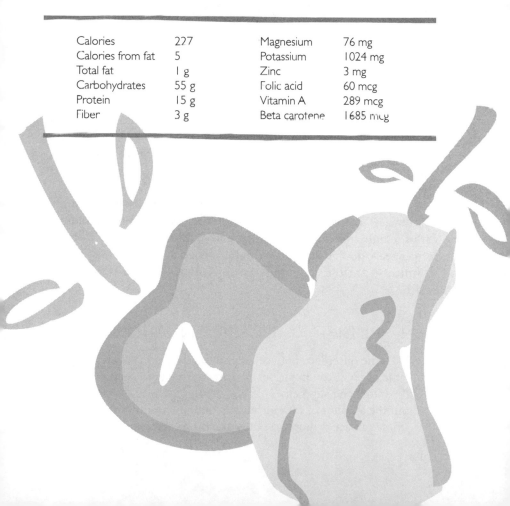

Calories	227	Magnesium	76 mg
Calories from fat	5	Potassium	1024 mg
Total fat	1 g	Zinc	3 mg
Carbohydrates	55 g	Folic acid	60 mcg
Protein	15 g	Vitamin A	289 mcg
Fiber	3 g	Beta carotene	1685 mcg

7

Rejuvenators

Smoothies for Youthful Skin

*Y*our skin is one of the most unforgiving organs. Every youthful indiscretion can leave its mark: deep dermal crevasses from smoking; crow's-feet from too many suntans; broken veins from alcohol; and dry skin from poor diet. And of course we cannot forget the effects of gravity or the toll of pollution.

The skin is one of the first organs to show the signs of nutrient deficiencies. Rejuvenate your skin from the inside out by providing it with the nutrients it needs to repair and maintain itself. Some of these recipes serve double duty: they can be applied externally as natural skin treatments. A clear, luminous skin has always been a sign of good health.

GENERAL DIETARY RECOMMENDATIONS

What's the difference between a plum and a prune? Water. Drink at least eight to ten glasses of water each day to keep your skin hydrated and supple.

Limit the amount of caffeine and alcohol in your diet. Both of these can act as diuretics, causing you to become dehydrated.

Eat a minimum of five servings a day of fruits and vegetables. These foods are rich in a wide variety of antioxidant compounds that will protect your skin from aging free radicals.

Substitute whole grain products for refined grains: eat brown bread instead of white, and eat brown rice instead of white. Whole grains are an important source of antioxidants and silicon needed for the manufacture of collagen and elastin, which give skin its youthful suppleness.

SMOOTHIE INGREDIENTS FOR YOUTHFUL SKIN

Avocados

The avocado contains between 20 and 30 percent fat. It is rich in vitamin E, which makes it a great skin moisturizer and conditioner when eaten or applied externally.

Brewer's Yeast

These microorganisms are one of the best sources of the B complex vitamins, chromium, and selenium. Chromium is necessary for healthy microcirculation of the skin, and selenium acts as an antioxidant that protects the skin cells from free radical damage. Brewer's yeast is considered in modern folklore to be an excellent facial scrub. Buy selenium-enriched brewer's yeast.

Flavonoids

The bioflavonoids are a family of substances with antioxidant abilities. They fortify skin tissue so that it is not as vulnerable to pollution, solar radiation, and other sources of free radicals. Bioflavonoids also strengthen the fine capillaries often seen broken in the skin. Bioflavonoids are found in citrus fruits, berries, and green and black tea.

Papayas

This carotene-rich fruit contains the protein-digesting enzyme papain. Since papain is destroyed by heat, only fresh papaya is a source of papain. Papaya puree makes a gentle facial exfoliant.

Peanut Butter

Peanuts are rich in protein, antioxidants, vitamin E, chromium, and the essential fatty acid linoleic acid—all nutrients essential to proper skin conditioning. When applied topically, peanut butter makes an effective moisturizing facial mask.

Pineapples

Pineapple is the source of bromelain, another protein-digesting enzyme. Bromelain is a natural anti-inflammatory agent and is destroyed by heat, so always use fresh pineapple when possible. Fresh pineapple can also be used as a facial exfoliant, to renew the surface layer of skin cells.

Protein

Protein provides the amino acids necessary for tissue regeneration. You can add protein to your smoothies by adding a scoop of protein powder or a cup of milk, soy milk, or yogurt.

Vitamin A

This fat-soluble vitamin is necessary for the health of epithelial cells, such as the epidermal layer of the skin. The best form of vitamin A is the provitamin A: beta carotene. This form is nontoxic and is present in most yellow, orange, and red fruits and vegetables.

Vitamin C

Vitamin C (ascorbic acid) when consumed or applied topically is a water-soluble antioxidant that protects cells from wrinkle-inducing free radical damage. Vitamin C is also necessary for the manufacture of collagen for the skin and connective tissue. You can add vitamin C to your smoothie as a powder. Guava, papaya, strawberries, citrus fruit, and tomato juice all will add vitamin C to your smoothie. When applied topically to the face, vitamin C has been shown to reduce the appearance of fine surface wrinkles.

Yogurt

In addition to calcium and protein, this fermented milk product is full of disease-fighting substances, including lactic acid and acetic acid, as well as an antibiotic dubbed acildopilin. Externally, yogurt is traditionally used to whiten and soften skin.

The Renovator

Papaya is a source of vitamin E, papain, and essential fatty acids, which makes it a perfect facial mask.

1 1/2 cups fresh papaya slices

1 teaspoon (about 500 mg) vitamin C powder

1 orange, peeled and seeded

1/2 cup nonfat milk

To make the facial mask, blend the papaya slices and vitamin C powder. Remove 1/2 cup of the mixture to use for the mask. Apply the mask to your skin and leave on for about 15 minutes.

Meanwhile, to make the smoothie, add the orange and milk to the remaining puree in the blender. Blend until smooth. Pour the smoothie into a glass and drink while the mask dries.

Calories	159	Calcium	236 mg
Calories from fat	5	Potassium	799 mg
Total fat	1 g	Folic acid	99 mcg
Carbohydrates	35 g	Vitamin C	492 mg
Protein	6 g	Vitamin A	384 mcg
Fiber	6 g		

Short Blonde Bombshell

The bromelain in pineapple acts as a skin exfoliant, removing dead skin and renewing the skin surface. The vitamin C added to this drink will help to reduce the appearance of fine wrinkles.

1 1/2 cups fresh or frozen pineapple chunks

1 tablespoon brewer's yeast

1 teaspoon (about 500 mg) vitamin C powder

1/2 cup nonfat milk

1 frozen banana, cut into pieces

1 tablespoon shredded coconut

To make the facial mask, blend 1 cup of the pineapple, brewer's yeast, and vitamin C powder. Remove 1/2 cup of the mixture to use for the mask. Apply the mask to your skin and leave on for about 15 minutes.

Meanwhile, add the milk, the remaining pineapple, banana, and coconut to the blender. Blend until smooth. Pour the smoothie into a glass and drink while the mask dries.

Calories	280	Iron	2 mg
Calories from fat	45	Niacin	3 mg
Total fat	5 g	Vitamin B6	1 mg
Carbohydrates	56 g	Folic acid	203 mcg
Protein	8 g	Vitamin C	288 mg
Fiber	6 g		

Kiwi Lemon Cream

The kiwifruit adds vitamin C and a protein-digesting enzyme. Yogurt and lemon juice are traditionally used to lighten and soften skin.

1 cup plain whole yogurt

1/2 lemon, peeled and seeded

2 kiwifruits, cut in half and the flesh scooped out

1 cup flavored nonfat frozen yogurt

To make the facial mask, blend the yogurt, lemon, and the flesh of one kiwifruit. Remove half of the mixture to use for the mask. Apply the mask to your skin and leave on for about 15 minutes.

Meanwhile, to make the smoothie, add the frozen yogurt and the remaining kiwifruit flesh to the remaining puree in the blender. Blend until smooth. Pour the smoothie into a glass and drink while the mask dries.

Calories	363	Calcium	331 mg
Calories from fat	38	Magnesium	65 mg
Total fat	4 g	Potassium	954 mg
Carbohydrates	70 g	Zinc	1 mg
Protein	13 g	Vitamin C	120 mg
Fiber	4 g		

Nutty Smile

The oils in peanut butter make it a perfect facial treatment.
Honey has been used for thousands of years to heal the skin.

1/4 cup smooth natural-style peanut butter

2 tablespoons honey

2 tablespoons plain nonfat yogurt

100 mg vitamin C powder

1 cup nonfat milk of choice

1 cup frozen strawberries

1 to 2 tablespoons orange juice concentrate

To make the facial mask, blend the peanut butter, honey, yogurt,
and vitamin C powder. Remove half of the mixture to use for the
mask. Apply the mask to your skin and leave on for about 15
minutes.

Meanwhile, to make the smoothie, add the milk, strawberries, and orange juice concentrate to the remaining puree in the
blender. Blend until smooth. Pour the smoothie into a glass and
drink while the mask dries.

Calories	420	Calcium	365 mg
Calories from fat	155	Magnesium	103 mg
Total fat	17 g	Folic acid	93 mcg
Carbohydrates	53 g	Vitamin C	160 mg
Protein	18 g	Vitamin A	162 mcg
Fiber	5 g	Vitamin E	3 mg

Avocado Freeze

Avocados add a buttery texture to smoothies as well as heart-healthy monounsaturated fats. Its oils will smooth and soften irritated skin while its vitamin E content heals.

1/2 avocado, pitted, peeled, and sliced

1 tablespoon lemon juice

1 cup frozen cherries, pitted

1 cup orange juice

To make the facial mask, blend the avocado and lemon juice. Remove half of the mixture to use for the mask. Apply the mask to your skin and leave on for about 15 minutes.

Meanwhile, to make the smoothie, add the cherries and orange juice to the remaining puree in the blender. Blend until smooth. Pour the smoothie into a glass and drink while the mask dries.

Calories	295	Niacin	2 mg
Calories from fat	81	Folic acid	145 mcg
Total fat	9 g	Vitamin C	114 mg
Carbohydrates	55 g	Vitamin A	76 mcg
Protein	4 g	Vitamin E	1 mg
Fiber	6 g		

Tahini Shake

The tahini (ground sesame seeds) adds a slightly nutty flavor to this thick shake.

1/2 cup nonfat milk

1 cup orange juice

1 frozen banana, cut into pieces

2 tablespoons tahini (ground sesame seeds)

Calories	438	Iron	3 mg
Calories from fat	153	Zinc	2 mg
Total fat	17 g	Folic acid	167 mcg
Carbohydrates	66 g	Vitamin C	108 mg
Protein	12 g	Vitamin E	2 mg
Fiber	6 g		

Berry Citrus Cup

This smoothie is full of vitamin C and anythocyanins, the red-to-blue flavonols that aid in building healthy skin tissue.

1 cup frozen blackberries

1 orange, peeled and seeded

1/2 cup orange juice

1/2 grapefruit, peeled and seeded

Calories	231	Magnesium	64 mg
Calories from fat	8	Potassium	923 mg
Total fat	1 g	Folic acid	155 mcg
Carbohydrates	57 g	Vitamin C	190 mg
Protein	4 g	Vitamin E	2 mg
Fiber	12 g		

Spotted Cot

The tiny seeds of the kiwifruit add interesting spots to this smoothie.

1 cup drained canned apricots

2 kiwifruits, cut in half and the flesh scooped out

1/2 cup plain nonfat yogurt

Calories	236	Iron	1 mg
Calories from fat	8	Zinc	2 mg
Total fat	1 g	Vitamin C	158 mg
Carbohydrates	52 g	Vitamin A	312 mcg
Protein	9 g	Beta carotene	1726 mcg
Fiber	8 g	Vitamin E	3 mg

Snappy Cot

The ginger in this smoothie is a natural anti-inflammatory agent.

1 1/2 cups drained canned apricots

1 cup vanilla nonfat yogurt

1 (1-inch) piece fresh ginger root, peeled
and crushed

Calories	338	Calcium	490 mg
Calories from fat	7	Zinc	2 mg
Total fat	1 g	Vitamin A	431 mcg
Carbohydrates	70 g	Beta carotene	2490 mcg
Protein	15 g	Vitamin E	2 mg
Fiber	4 g		

Peanut Butter Shake

For a meal replacement, add a scoop or two of protein powder to this drink.

1 frozen banana, cut into pieces

1 cup milk of choice

1/4 cup natural-style peanut butter

1 teaspoon cinnamon

Calories	573	Iron	2 mg
Calories from fat	297	Zinc	3 mg
Total fat	33 g	Niacin	9 mg
Carbohydrates	54 g	Vitamin B6	1 mg
Protein	25 g	Vitamin E	7 mg
Fiber	8 g		

Strawberry in Heaven

Berries contain flavonoids that help to build the strong connective tissue necessary for healthy skin.

1 cup frozen strawberries

1/2 cup whole soy milk

1/2 cup vanilla nonfat yogurt

2 tablespoons vanilla protein powder

1 tablespoon flaxseed powder

Calories	295	Calcium	333 mg
Calories from fat	63	Iron	6 mg
Total fat	7 g	Magnesium	84 mg
Carbohydrates	33 g	Zinc	2 mg
Protein	30 g	Vitamin C	85 mg
Fiber	6 g		

Lovely Linda

For a thicker smoothie, use frozen pineapple.

1 cup drained canned peaches

3/4 cup fresh pineapple chunks

1/4 cup plain nonfat yogurt

1 tablespoon brewer's yeast

Calories	195	Iron	2 mg
Calories from fat	7	Niacin	5 mg
Total fat	1 g	Thiamin	1 mg
Carbohydrates	43 g	Folic acid	336 mcg
Protein	8 g	Vitamin E	3 mg
Fiber	4 g		

Orange Berry Screamer

Vitamins, minerals, and protein—this smoothie has it all.

1 1/2 cups frozen strawberries

1 cup orange juice

1 tablespoon vanilla protein powder

1 teaspoon flaxseed oil

1 teaspoon brewer's yeast

Calories	260	Iron	2 mg
Calories from fat	52	Thiamin	0.7 mg
Total fat	6 g	Folic acid	252 mcg
Carbohydrates	44 g	Vitamin C	224 mg
Protein	13 g	Vitamin E	3 mg
Fiber	6 g		

CHAPTER 8

Soothers

Smoothies for Stress Reduction

S tress is a major by-product of the nineties lifestyle. We are under physical stress from environmental pollution, physical trauma, and a fast-food diet and mental stress from the often colliding obligations of work, family, and finances. In our bodies, these strains trigger the stress response.

The adrenal glands produce the hormones responsible for the stress response. Epinephrine and norepinephrine are produced by the inner portion of the adrenal gland, and the corticosteroids are produced by the outer layer. These hormones allow the body to prepare itself for vigorous physical exertion. For example, when epinephrine levels in the blood rise in response to stress, this stimulates the heart, constricts the small arterioles, raises the blood pressure, frees sugar stored in the liver, and relaxes certain involuntary muscles while contracting others.

Blood is diverted from unneeded areas such as the digestive system and sent to the muscles and heart. In the case of the gastrointestinal tract, the stomach empties itself by vomiting and the colon by diarrhea. Food in the small intestine that cannot be expelled is held until normal functioning returns. After the body returns to normal, the nutrients depleted in the production of the adrenal hormones must be replaced, or shortages can occur.

GENERAL DIETARY RECOMMENDATIONS

Eat a whole foods diet rich in whole grains and fruits and vegetables. The fiber will help to decrease cholesterol levels increased by the stress and temper the constipation and diarrhea caused by stress.

During periods of stress, avoid heavy fatty foods and substitute easy-to-digest lowfat choices. The stress response increases blood flow to the muscles while pulling blood away from the-digestive tract. This causes a reduction in gastric and intestinal secretions necessary for digestion.

Reduce your consumption of caffeine-containing beverages, such as coffee, tea, and colas. This stimulant only increases the stress on your body.

Avoid alcohol. Beer, wine, and spirits may appear to offer short-term relief, but they only further deplete your system resources.

Decrease your sodium intake. The aldosterone produced by the stressed adrenal gland causes sodium retention.

SMOOTHIE INGREDIENTS FOR STRESS REDUCTION

Brewer's Yeast

Brewer's yeast contains B-complex vitamins, which are depleted in times of physical and emotional stress. Vitamin B6 (pyridoxine) deficiency is often found in depressed people, and some studies have shown that mood improves when vitamin B6 supplements are given. Pantothenic acid is necessary to replenish cortisone depleted by the stress response.

Calcium

This mineral stimulates muscles and contracts blood vessels. Mild calcium deficiency can cause nerve sensitivity, muscle twitching, irritability, and insomnia. When blood calcium levels drop below normal, the sensitivity of the nerves can increase, leading to muscle cramps. Milk, yogurt, fortified soy milk, and orange juice are sources of calcium that can be added to smoothies.

Lecithin

Choline is a component of the neurotransmitter acetylcholine, which is involved in many nerve and brain functions; dietary intake of choline seems to affect body levels of acetylcholine. Choline is an active ingredient in lecithin. It is a component of cell membranes and of myelin, the insulating sheath around the nerves. Lecithin granules can be added to smoothies.

Magnesium

This mineral is a natural tranquilizer that acts in conjunction with calcium. Magnesium relaxes skeletal muscle of the arms and legs as well as smooth muscle in the digestive tract and circulatory system. When magnesium levels are too low, more calcium flows into muscle cells, causing them to contract. This mechanism can increase blood pressure or cause muscle cramps. The adrenaline secreted by the adrenal gland during stress increases urinary excretion of magnesium. Magnesium deficiency then stimulates stress hormones, further aggravating the stress response, which results in depression and irritability. Since magnesium competes for absorption with calcium, a high calcium intake may lead to magnesium deficiency. Magnesium is available as a liquid in health food stores. Or you can use bananas, blueberries, carrot juice, cherries, dates, grapefruit, oranges, tomato juice, and raspberries to add magnesium to your smoothies.

Potassium

The excretion of this mineral is increased by the corticosteroids produced by the adrenal glands during the stress response. Bananas and cantaloupes are good sources of potassium. Many liquid herbal formulas contain added potassium.

Psyllium Seed

When the body is stressed, cholesterol levels remain elevated. Some types of fiber can help to decrease cholesterol levels by binding with the cholesterol in bile salts in the colon before they can be reabsorbed. This increases the amount of cholesterol excreted. In one study, participants took one teaspoon of psyllium seed powder three times a day for eight weeks. This resulted in a significant decrease in blood cholesterol levels.

Vitamin C

This antioxidant is necessary to replenish the hormones depleted by the stress response. Strawberries, papayas, to-mato juice, and citrus fruits are rich in vitamin C as well as potassium.

Zinc

Zinc is an antioxidant mineral that is necessary to replenish the hormones depleted by the stress response. Nuts, seeds, and whole grains are good sources of zinc.

HERBS FOR STRESS REDUCTION

Ginseng

In naturopathic medicine, ginseng is defined as an adaptogen: an agent that protects against stress and normalizes an abnormal state. The ginsenosides in ginseng maintain homeostasis and improves adrenal gland function.

Kava

Kava is an herb used for the relief of short-term stress and depression. Kava root extract is the herbal equivalent of Valium and Xanax. In Europe, it is used to reduce anxiety without decreasing mental awareness.

Yogi Smoothie

Here's an unusual drink, based on Indian spices.

1 cup skim milk
1 cup frozen nonfat yogurt
1 tablespoon sweetener
1/2 teaspoon ground cinnamon
1/4 teaspoon ground cloves
1/4 teaspoon ground ginger
1/4 teaspoon ground cardamom
Pinch ground black pepper

Calories	379	Calcium	484 mg
Calories from fat	5	Magnesium	49 mg
Total fat	1 g	Zinc	2 mg
Carbohydrates	77 g	Riboflavin	1 mg
Protein	17 g	Vitamin B12	3 mcg
Fiber	1 g		

Honeyed Orange

Honey has been used as a sleeping aid for hundreds of years.

1 cup orange juice

1 banana

2 tablespoons honey

200 mg vitamin C powder

Calories	347	Magnesium	59 mg
Calories from fat	6	Potassium	947 mg
Total fat	1 g	Vitamin B6	1 mg
Carbohydrates	88 g	Folic acid	133 mcg
Protein	3 g	Vitamin C	307 mg
Fiber	3 g		

Pineapple Date

A combination of three fruits, which when eaten on an empty stomach increase insulin levels. When insulin levels rise, more tryptophan can enter the brain, to make you sleepy.

1 1/2 cups pineapple juice

1 banana

1/4 cup soaked dates

Calories	411	Iron	2 mg
Calories from fat	9	Magnesium	97 mg
Total fat	1 g	Niacin	2 mg
Carbohydrates	105 g	Vitamin B6	1 mg
Protein	3 g	Folic acid	113 mcg
Fiber	5 g		

Cherry Shake

This smoothie contains the fiber needed to assure regularity during times of stress. The psyllium seed will also help to decrease the elevated cholesterol levels that occur during stress.

1 cup frozen cherries

1 banana

1 cup nonfat milk

1 teaspoon psyllium seed powder

Calories	295	Calcium	331 mg
Calories from fat	22	Magnesium	77 mg
Total fat	2 g	Potassium	1212 mg
Carbohydrates	66 g	Riboflavin	1 mg
Protein	11 g	Vitamin B6	1 mg
Fiber	10 g		

Banana Snap

This drink provides lecithin, to replenish the choline used during the stress response.

1 cup orange juice

1 frozen banana, cut into pieces

1 (1/2-inch) piece fresh ginger root, peeled and crushed

1 tablespoon lecithin granules

1 teaspoon brewer's yeast

Calories	344	Magnesium	66 mg
Calories from fat	131	Potassium	1062 mg
Total fat	15 g	Niacin	2 mg
Carbohydrates	58 g	Folic acid	234 mcg
Protein	4 g	Vitamin C	108 mg
Fiber	3 g		

Cherry Dream

The magnesium in this smoothie will help to relax tense muscles.

1 cup vanilla nonfat yogurt

1 cup frozen cherries

Powdered magnesium supplement (see label for recommended dosage)

Calories	292	Calcium	474 mg
Calories from fat	16	Magnesium	59 mg
Total fat	2 g	Potassium	904 mg
Carbohydrates	57 g	Zinc	2 mg
Protein	15 g	Riboflavin	1 mg
Fiber	3 g		

Orange Soother

Rich in potassium and vitamin C, this drink is a great way to restore needed nutrients after a stressful day.

1 cup fresh carrot juice

1/2 cup orange juice

1/2 cup mango slices

1/2 cup ice

Calories	208	Potassium	1086 mg
Calories from fat	6	Vitamin B6	1 mg
Total fat	1 g	Folic acid	76 mcg
Carbohydrates	50 g	Vitamin C	92 mg
Protein	4 g	Vitamin A	6666 mcg
Fiber	4 g	Beta carotene	24443 mcg

Nutty Blonde

Peanut butter goes well with the sweet taste of pineapple.

1 1/2 cups pineapple

1 frozen banana, cut into pieces

2 tablespoons natural-style peanut butter

1 tablespoon lecithin granules

Calories	513	Iron	2 mg
Calories from fat	280	Magnesium	113 mg
Total fat	31 g	Niacin	6 mg
Carbohydrates	62 g	Folic acid	71 mcg
Protein	10 g	Vitamin E	4 mg
Fiber	7 g		

Orange Froth

Brewer's yeast and banana add pyridoxine (vitamin B6), which can improve your mood when stress gets you down.

1 1/2 cups orange juice

1 frozen banana, cut into pieces

1 tablespoon lecithin granules

1 teaspoon brewer's yeast

Calories	385	Magnesium	69 mg
Calories from fat	130	Niacin	2 mg
Total fat	14 g	Vitamin B6	1 mg
Carbohydrates	68 g	Folic Acid	289 mcg
Protein	5 g	Vitamin C	156 mg
Fiber	4 g		

Ginseng Soother

Ginseng has been used for centuries as an adaptogen, a substance that helps an organism to adapt to stressful circumstances.

2 kiwifruits, cut in half and flesh scooped out

1 cup orange juice

1/2 cup ice

Ginseng supplement (see label for
    recommended dosage)

Calories	204	Magnesium	71 mg
Calories from fat	7	Potassium	979 mg
Total fat	1 g	Folic acid	167 mcg
Carbohydrates	50 g	Vitamin C	246 mg
Protein	3 g	Vitamin E	2 mg
Fiber	6 g		

Tropical Tahini

Here's a good way to replenish the potassium, magnesium, and other minerals lost during the day.

1 cup mango slices

1 cup fresh or canned pineapple, drained

1/4 cup guava nectar

2 tablespoons tahini

Powdered or liquid magnesium supplement
   (see label for recommended dosage)

Calories	402	Iron	3 mg
Calories from fat	155	Niacin	3 mg
Total fat	17 g	Vitamin C	85 mg
Carbohydrates	63 g	Beta carotene	621 mcg
Protein	7 g	Vitamin E	3 mg
Fiber	8 g		

Blue Hurricane

The mild flavor of this smoothie takes the addition of heavily flavored herbal supplements well.

1 1/2 cups frozen blueberries

1 banana

Liquid herbal extract (see label for
recommended dosage)

Calories	227	Magnesium	44 mg
Calories from fat	13	Potassium	645 mg
Total fat	1 g	Niacin	1 mg
Carbohydrates	57 g	Vitamin B6	1 mg
Protein	3 g	Vitamin E	2 mg
Fiber	9 g		

Dreamy Lisa

Full of magnesium and calcium, this drink will nourish irritated nerves and aid in relaxation.

1 1/2 cups vanilla nonfat yogurt

1 1/2 cups frozen blueberries

Powdered magnesium supplement (see label for recommended dosage)

Kava root extract (see label for recommended dosage)

Calories	404	Calcium	691 mg
Calories from fat	13	Magnesium	75 mg
Total fat	1 g	Zinc	4 mg
Carbohydrates	80 g	Riboflavin	1 mg
Protein	21 g	Vitamin E	2 mg
Fiber	6 g		

Libido Enhancers

Smoothies to Strengthen the Reproductive System

*I*t is said that the brain is the most important sexual organ. There-fore it follows that any stresses on nerve and brain function will eventually also affect your love life. Equipment maintenance is also im-portant. The most common physical cause of male sexual dysfunction is damage to blood vessels, which impairs blood flow to the penis. This is usually caused by atherosclerosis.

A new Finnish study has shown that middle-aged and older men have become significantly less fertile. They found not only a drop in sperm quality over the last fifty years but also an increasing number of problems with male reproductive organs, including a decrease in the size of the seminiferous tubules, a decrease in the weight of the testi-cles, and an increase in the amount of fibrotic tissue. At least some of these changes may be due to a poor diet and the need for more anti-oxidants because of pollution.

GENERAL DIETARY RECOMMENDATIONS

Men should follow a heart-healthy diet that is low in saturated fat and high in complex carbohydrates. This will help to reduce the atherosclerosis that can decrease blood flow to the penis. The typical Western diet, which is high in fat, may be linked to low testosterone levels.

Eliminate caffeine from your diet. Caffeine in coffee and soda (but not in tea) was linked to a decrease in fertility. In one study, one caffeinated soft drink was enough to decrease fertility by 50 percent.

SMOOTHIE INGREDIENTS TO ENHANCE FERTILITY

Antioxidants

Antioxidants protect the membranes of the sperm from oxygen free radical damage. This damage lowers the sperm's ability to recognize and penetrate the egg. Orange, yellow, and red fruits and vegetables and citrus fruits can be added to smoothies to increase their antioxidant levels.

Brewer's Yeast

The B vitamins folacin and pyridoxine (vitamin B6) may be lower in women who have taken oral contraceptives. Brewer's yeast is an excellent source of all the B vitamins. Add one tablespoon to any smoothie.

Copper

This trace element may be involved in the maturation of sperm and is part of an enzyme that neutralizes free radicals that may cause infertility. Copper is often included in protein mixes.

Vitamin E

This fat-soluble vitamin may help men to increase their fertilization rates. In one study of normal males with low fertilization rates, the chances of conception were increased 10 percent by 200 mg/day of vitamin E. Liquid vitamin E can be added to smoothies. Wheat germ and almonds also increase the vitamin E content of smoothies. Peanut butter is another source of vitamin E.

SMOOTHIE INGREDIENTS TO ENHANCE SEXUAL FUNCTION

L-Arginine

Arginine is an amino acid that may enhance male sexual function. This may be due to its ability to increase circulation by dilating the arteries. Indirectly, arginine is related to sperm production. A powdered form of arginine can be purchased in health food stores.

Chocolate

Chocolate and cocoa contain three substances from the chemical group N-acelethanolamine. These substances stimulate the area of the brain that produces feelings of pleasure and are similar to the chemicals found in marijuana. One of these substances, phenylethylalamine, is made naturally when in love and during the sexual act. Chocolate and cocoa also contain theobromide, a mild stimulant.

Tyrosine and Phenylalanine

These two amino acids are the precursors to many of the sexual arousal and response neurotransmitters, including norepinephrine and dopamine. A deficiency of phenylalanine can lead to depression and a lack of sexual drive. Tyrosine can be purchased in powdered form and added to smoothies.

Vanilla

Pure vanilla extract has a stimulating effect on the motor nerves used in sexual response.

Vitamin A

This fat-soluble vitamin is necessary for the growth and repair of epithelial cells. Epithelial cells cover the parts of the body that come into contact with the outside world, such as the skin, the digestive tract, the urinary system, and the reproductive organs. Therefore it is important in the maintenance of the lining of the vagina and uterus. Vitamin A is manufactured by the body from the orange pigment beta carotene. Good smoothie additions are papayas, mangos, peaches, apricots, cantaloupes, pink grapefruits, and carrot juice.

Vitamin E

This fat-soluble vitamin may have libido-enhancing properties. Studies show that daily intake of vitamin E delays testosterone breakdown, thereby sustaining its effects over a longer period of time. Vitamin E can be added to smoothies as a liquid. Wheat germ and almonds also increase the vitamin E content of smoothies.

Zinc

Zinc is necessary for fertility, potency, and sexual drive. Zinc deficiency can lead to reduced sperm production, lower semen, and testosterone levels. Pumpkin seed butter is a rich source of vegetarian zinc that can be added to smoothies. Wheat germ, oatmeal, and soybeans also contain zinc in smaller quantities.

HERBS TO ENHANCE FERTILITY AND SEXUAL FUNCTION

Ginseng

In the East, this herb is widely prized for its legendary aphrodisiac properties. In the West, research concerning its use for this intent is still controversial. Ginseng strengthens the heart and nervous system, increases the body's hormone production, stimulates metabolism, prevents fatigue and the aging phenomenon, and aids against stresses through stimulation of the cerebrocortical functions.

Licorice

Licorice root contains chemicals related to adrenal and ovarian secretions, such as mineralocorticoid-like substances, beta-sitosterol, and stigmasterol. Their estrogenic activity supports licorice's use as a uterine tonic and as a fertility enhancer.

Fuzzy Navel

Peachy and fresh tasting, this smoothie contains tyrosine, an amino acid needed to produce neurotransmitters necessary for sexual arousal.

1 cup orange juice

1/2 cup vanilla lowfat yogurt

2 peaches, pitted and peeled, or 4 canned peach halves, drained

1 frozen banana, cut into pieces

1 tablespoon flaxseed powder

Tyrosine supplement (see label for recommended dosage)

Calories	438	Iron	5 mg
Calories from fat	51	Magnesium	109 mg
Total fat	6 g	Niacin	3 mg
Carbohydrates	92 g	Folic acid	149 mcg
Protein	12 g	Vitamin C	120 mg
Fiber	8 g		

Apple Libation

Double this recipe and serve it with two straws.

1 cup lime sorbet

2 apples, cored, peeled, and sliced

3 tablespoons honey

1 tablespoon lime juice

1 (2-inch) piece fresh ginger, peeled and crushed

Ginseng supplement (see label for
   recommended dosage)

Calories	655	Fiber	6 g
Calories from fat	13	Iron	1 mg
Total fat	1 g	Magnesium	48 mg
Carbohydrates	165 g	Potassium	694 mg
Protein	3 g	Niacin	1 mg

Heart's Desire

The fruits and wheat germ in this smoothie are full of anti-oxidants, which help to protect the sperm from free radical damage.

1/2 cup purple grape juice

1 cup frozen cherries

1 cup black cherry nonfat yogurt

1 frozen banana, cut into pieces

1 tablespoon flaxseed powder

1 tablespoon wheat germ

Calories	586	Calcium	398 mg
Calories from fat	73	Iron	7 mg
Total fat	8 g	Magnesium	112 mg
Carbohydrates	119 g	Zinc	2 mg
Protein	18 g	Folic acid	363 mcg
Fiber	7 g		

Almond Cream

Fragrant with the aroma of vanilla, this smoothie is a good source of the B vitamins, which may be deficient in women on oral contraceptives.

1 cup almond milk

1/2 cup soft or silken tofu

1 frozen banana, cut into pieces

1 tablespoon brewer's yeast

3 drops pure vanilla extract

Calories	488	Iron	6 mg
Calories from fat	268	Magnesium	171 mg
Total fat	30 g	Thiamin	1 mg
Carbohydrates	36 g	Folic acid	362 mcg
Protein	22 g	Vitamin E	11 mg
Fiber	3 g		

Chocolate Stimulant

The cocoa in this drink contains phenylethylalamine, a substance made naturally when in love.

2 cups almond milk

1/2 cup ice

6 tablespoons cocoa powder

1 tablespoon brewer's yeast

Calories	680	Iron	9 mg
Calories from fat	473	Magnesium	427 mg
Total fat	53 g	Zinc	5 mg
Carbohydrates	25 g	Niacin	7 mg
Protein	27 g	Vitamin E	22 mg
Fiber	0 g		

Licorice Cooler

Licorice is a traditional fertility enhancer.

1 cup fortified soy milk

1 cup vanilla nonfat frozen yogurt or vanilla nonfat yogurt

Liquid licorice root extract (see label for recommended dosage)

Calories	322	Calcium	581 mg
Calories from fat	67	Magnesium	90 mg
Total fat	7 g	Zinc	3 mg
Carbohydrates	43 g	Beta carotene	410 mcg
Protein	21 g	Vitamin E	7 mg
Fiber	5 g		

Chocolate Nut

The vitamin E supplement adds to the vitamin E found in peanut butter.

1 cup nonfat milk

1 cup vanilla lowfat frozen yogurt

1/4 cup natural-style peanut butter

2 tablespoons cocoa protein powder

2 tablespoons chocolate syrup

Vitamin E supplement (see label for recommended dosage)

Calories	854	Calcium	504 mg
Calories from fat	319	Iron	3 mg
Total fat	35 g	Magnesium	163 mg
Carbohydrates	93 g	Zinc	4 mg
Protein	49 g	Vitamin A	150 mcg
Fiber	4 g	Vitamin E	6 mg

Divine Daiquiri

The flavonoids and vitamin C found in this recipe help to protect sperm from free radical damage.

1 cup lemon sorbet

1 lime, peeled and seeded

1 teaspoon honey

1 teaspoon flaxseed oil

Vitamin C powder (see label for recommended dosage)

Calories	332	Protein	1 g
Calories from fat	41	Fiber	2 g
Total fat	5 g	Vitamin E	2 mg
Carbohydrates	75 g		

Hindu Love Goddess

This sensual treat is a traditional stimulant.

1 cup nonfat milk

1 cup vanilla lowfat frozen yogurt

3 dates, pitted and chopped

1/8 teaspoon ground cloves

1/8 teaspoon ground cardamom

1/8 teaspoon ground cinnamon

1/4 teaspoon pure vanilla extract

Calories	395	Calcium	436 mg
Calories from fat	23	Iron	2 mg
Total fat	3 g	Magnesium	70 mg
Carbohydrates	76 g	Potassium	886 mg
Protein	15 g	Zinc	2 mg
Fiber	1 g		

Afterglow

Here's a unique, cool smoothie with the slight nutty taste of sesame.

1 cup vanilla soy milk

1/2 cup silken tofu

1/2 cup vanilla lowfat ice cream

1 tablespoon tahini (ground sesame seeds)

Calories	426	Calcium	328 mg
Calories from fat	209	Iron	5 mg
Total fat	23 g	Potassium	241 mg
Carbohydrates	37 g	Zinc	1 mg
Protein	19 g	Niacin	1 mg
Fiber	4 g		

Peach Heaven

Rich in vitamin A and soy isoflavones, this drink makes the perfect background for a licorice supplement.

1 cup drained canned peaches

1/2 cup whole soy milk

1/2 cup vanilla nonfat yogurt

2 tablespoons vanilla soy protein powder

1 tablespoon flaxseed powder

1 teaspoon pure vanilla extract

Licorice powder (see label for
    recommended dosage)

Calories	372	Calcium	328 mg
Calories from fat	59	Iron	6 mg
Total fat	7 g	Magnesium	87 mg
Carbohydrates	52 g	Zinc	2 mg
Protein	31 g	Vitamin E	4 mg
Fiber	6 g		

Ginseng Shake

Ginseng has been used in Asia for centuries as a sexual tonic.

1/2 cup nonfat milk

1/2 cup orange juice

1 frozen banana, cut into pieces

Liquid ginseng supplement (see label for recommended dosage)

Calories	204	Magnesium	59 mg
Calories from fat	7	Potassium	891 mg
Total fat	1 g	Niacin	1 mg
Carbohydrates	46 g	Vitamin B6	1 mg
Protein	6 g	Folic acid	83 mcg
Fiber	3 g		

Licorice Shake

This drink will reduce cholesterol levels. Atherosclerosis is a common cause of erection difficulties in men.

1 cup vanilla nonfat yogurt

1 frozen banana, cut into pieces

1 1/2 teaspoons pure vanilla extract

L-arginine (see label for recommended dosage)

Licorice extract (see label for
   recommended dosage)

1 teaspoon psyllium seed powder

Calories	311	Calcium	459 mg
Calories from fat	9	Magnesium	76 mg
Total fat	1 g	Potassium	1069 mg
Carbohydrates	64 g	Zinc	2 mg
Protein	14 g	Vitamin B6	0.8 mg
Fiber	6 g		

Burning Blue Jim

This drink is a spicy source of arginine—an amino acid that may enhance male sexual function.

1 cup frozen blueberries

1 cup frozen blackberries

1 cup berry nonfat yogurt

1 teaspoon ground cinnamon

1/2-inch piece crushed fresh ginger root

L-arginine (see label for recommended dosage)

Calories	390	Calcium	398 mg
Calories from fat	34	Iron	2 mg
Total fat	4 g	Zinc	2 mg
Carbohydrates	84 g	Vitamin C	51 mg
Protein	11 g	Vitamin E	2 mg
Fiber	13 g		

CHAPTER 10

Memory Boosters

Smoothies to Improve Cognitive Function

$\mathcal{M}$ emory formation is a complex biochemical process that is very poorly understood. To support memory and cognitive function, the brain must be furnished with the proper neurotransmitters and their cofactors, ample blood supply to deliver oxygen, and the nutrients, fatty acids, and fuel in the form of blood sugar. As people age, vitamin and mineral absorption becomes less efficient. Empty-nesters no longer feel the need to cook and serve balanced meals when they are cooking for only two. Together, these can result in nutrient deficiencies. Smoothies offer a quick, easy method of presenting your body with highly absorbable nutrients that can keep your memory sharp.

GENERAL DIETARY RECOMMENDATIONS

Need to memorize something? While studying, snack on a high-fat food. Fat stimulates the production of cholecystokinin, a neurotransmitter that may help to secure the information in your memory.

Rule out hypoglycemia by visiting your doctor for tests. Low blood sugar is infamous for causing brain fog.

MEMORY-BOOSTING SMOOTHIE INGREDIENTS

Acetyl-L-Carnitine

This form of the amino acid carnitine improves learning and memory in both cognitively impaired and normal humans of all ages and has been used for many years in Italy to treat Alzheimer's disease. Acetyl-L-Carnitine also elevates mood, alleviates depression, and improves cerebral blood flow. It is available in powdered form to add to smoothies.

Beta Carotene

This orange pigment may protect against memory impairment and the loss of mental function. In the new study of more than 5,100 people, those who consumed less than 0.9 milligrams per day of beta carotene were almost twice as likely to suffer memory impairment, disorientation, and difficulty solving problems as those who consumed 2.1 milligrams a day or more. Antioxidants have been implicated in processes related to atherosclerosis, aging, and selective neuronal damage, all of which may ultimately affect cognitive function. In another study, higher vitamin C and beta carotene levels were associated with higher scores on free recall, recognition, and vocabulary tests. Any orange-colored fruit, such as apricots, peaches, pumpkin puree, carrot juice, mangoes, and papayas, will add beta carotene to smoothies.

Boron

A research study with participants over forty-five years of age found that electrical activity was greater in subjects fed a high-boron diet. Those fed a low-boron diet took longer to perform the same cognitive tasks. You can increase the boron content of your smoothie by adding apples, pears, peaches, grapes, and peanut butter.

Brewer's Yeast

Thiamin (B1), riboflavin (B2), and pyridoxine (B6) lessen symptoms of depression and improve cognitive function in seniors. These B-complex vitamins are cofactors for the neurotransmitters involved with mood and cognitive function.

Folic acid

A deficiency of this B vitamin was linked to low scores on a memory test. Orange juice, wheat germ, and brewer's yeast will increase the folate content of smoothies.

Iron

Low iron levels in the brain may impair brain function by affecting the production and function of neurotransmitters. In one study of seventy-eight girls with mildly low iron levels (but not anemia), those who took iron supplements showed improvements on tests measuring their memory and their ability to recall new vocabulary words when compared with teens who were not given iron. Iron deficiency is more likely in teens who grow rapidly, teens who are vegetarian, and adolescent girls with heavy menstrual periods. Iron can be added to smoothies as part of a protein or multivitamin/mineral supplement. Prunes, raisins, and wheat germ will increase the iron content of smoothies.

Lecithin

Acetylcholine is a neurotransmitter that is important for memory in humans. It is made out of choline which the body also synthesizes. Under normal circumstances, the body does not need a dietary source of choline. However, when nerve cells are stressed the need for acetylcholine outpaces the rate at which choline can be manufactured. If dietary choline is not available, the body will even steal choline for the cell membranes to use in acetylcholine production. This results in membrane damage. Lecithin can be purchased in granular form and added to smoothies.

Vitamin B12

A deficiency in this vitamin has been linked with memory problems. Vitamin B12 is absorbed less efficiently as we age, and low levels are often found in vegans and those with stomach disorders. B12 can be added to smoothies as a supplement. Brewer's yeast is also a good source of this vitamin.

Vitamin C

A high intake of ascorbic acid (vitamin C) may protect against both cognitive impairment and cerebrovascular disease. In a nutritional survey, cognitive function was poorest in those with the lowest vitamin C status. High blood plasma levels of vitamin C and beta carotene were linked to better memory, according to researchers at the University of Bern. In a study of 442 men and women, higher vitamin C and beta carotene levels were associated with higher scores on free recall, recognition, and vocabulary tests.

MEMORY-BOOSTING HERBS

Ginkgo

The extract of this herb is used to enhance circulation and memory. A recent article in the *Journal of the American Medical Association* found *ginkgo biloba* extract to be safe and effective in improving the mental performance and social functioning of patients with Alzheimer's disease and dementia.

Memory Maker

This drink is rich in boron, choline, and vitamin C—all are nutrients needed for memory.

1 cup apple juice

1 cup orange juice

1/2 cup ice

1 tablespoon lecithin granules

1 teaspoon brewer's yeast

Ginkgo biloba extract (see label for
recommended dosage)

Calories	341	Iron	2 mg
Calories from fat	126	Niacin	2 mg
Total fat	14 g	Thiamin	1 mg
Carbohydrates	57 g	Folic acid	213 mcg
Protein	3 g	Vitamin C	99 mg
Fiber	1 g		

Sea Shake

This smoothie gets its iron from the algae.

1 cup soy milk

1 cup lowfat frozen yogurt

1 frozen banana, cut into pieces

2 tablespoons vanilla protein powder

1 teaspoon algae

Calories	506	Iron	5 mg
Calories from fat	73	Magnesium	122 mg
Total fat	8 g	Zinc	2 mg
Carbohydrates	78 g	Riboflavin	1 mg
Protein	34 g	Thiamin	1 mg
Fiber	6 g	Vitamin B6	1 mg

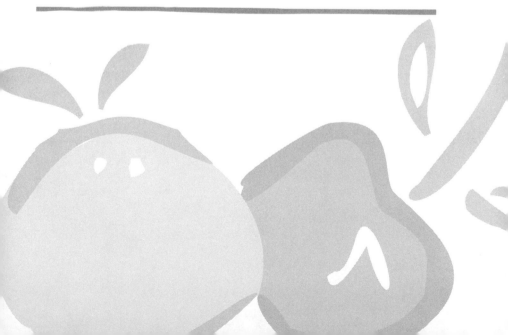

Orange Shake

Deficiencies of the B-complex vitamins are often the cause of poor cognitive function. This recipe brings B6 from the banana, B12 from the yeast, and folate from the orange.

1/2 cup whole soy milk

1 frozen banana, cut into pieces

1 orange, peeled and seeded

1 tablespoon brewer's yeast

1 tablespoon wheat germ

Calories	258	Iron	3 mg
Calories from fat	34	Niacin	5 mg
Total fat	4 g	Thiamin	2 mg
Carbohydrates	51 g	Vitamin B6	1 mg
Protein	10 g	Folic acid	397 mcg
Fiber	9 g		

Super Sipper

Here's the perfect drink to increase your brain power. The absorption of iron in the prunes and wheat germ is enhanced by the vitamin C in the strawberries.

1 cup frozen strawberries

1/2 cup prune juice

1 frozen banana, cut into pieces

1 tablespoon wheat germ

1 tablespoon lecithin granules

1 teaspoon brewer's yeast

200 to 300 mg vitamin C powder

Calories	457	Iron	5 mg
Calories from fat	158	Magnesium	136 mg
Total fat	18 g	Zinc	4 mg
Carbohydrates	76 g	Vitamin B6	1 mg
Protein	11 g	Folic acid	234 mcg
Fiber	12 g	Vitamin E	5 mg

Peachy Keane

Peaches are a wonderful source of beta carotene.

1 cup orange juice

1 cup drained canned peaches

2 tablespoons vanilla protein powder

1 teaspoon brewer's yeast

Calories	297	Niacin	3 mg
Calories from fat	8	Thiamin	1 mg
Total fat	1 g	Folic acid	217 mcg
Carbohydrates	57 g	Vitamin C	106 mg
Protein	22 g	Vitamin E	4 mg
Fiber	4 g		

Fruit Cup with Frost on Top

This form of the amino acid carnitine improves learning and memory.

1 cup drained canned peaches

1/2 cup frozen strawberries

1/2 cup orange juice

Powdered Acetyl-L-Carnitine (see label for recommended dosage)

2 tablespoons lemon sorbet for garnish

Calories	219	Potassium	677 mg
Calories from fat	4	Niacin	2 mg
Total fat	0 g	Folic acid	72 mcg
Carbohydrates	55 g	Vitamin C	100 mg
Protein	3 g	Vitamin E	4 mg
Fiber	5 g		

Strawberry Froth

This smoothie is a frothy blend of vitamin C, folate, and choline.

1 cup frozen strawberries

1 cup orange juice

1 banana

1 tablespoon lecithin granules

Calories	366	Magnesium	73 mg
Calories from fat	133	Potassium	1172 mg
Total fat	15 g	Vitamin B6	1 mg
Carbohydrates	64 g	Folic acid	157 mcg
Protein	4 g	Vitamin C	192 mg
Fiber	7 g		

Prune Shake

Wheat germ and prunes supply the iron, and apple juice supplies the boron in this mineral-rich drink.

1 cup apple juice

1/2 cup pureed prunes

1 frozen banana, cut into pieces

1 tablespoon wheat germ

200 mg vitamin C powder

Calories	338	Iron	2 mg
Calories from fat	16	Zinc	1 mg
Total fat	2 g	Niacin	2 mg
Carbohydrates	83 g	Vitamin B6	1 mg
Protein	4 g	Vitamin C	217 mg
Fiber	6 g		

Study Buddy

Sip this calorie-rich smoothie while you study, to help you retain more of what you read.

1 cup frozen strawberries

1 cup vanilla nonfat yogurt

3 tablespoons chocolate sauce

3 tablespoons peanut butter

1 tablespoon lecithin granules

1 teaspoon flaxseed oil

Calories	786	Calcium	499 mg
Calories from fat	392	Iron	3 mg
Total fat	44 g	Zinc	4 mg
Carbohydrates	86 g	Riboflavin	1 mg
Protein	27 g	Niacin	7 mg
Fiber	6 g	Vitamin E	6 mg

Pink Hurricane

The antioxidants in the raspberries will complement any herbs you add to this smoothie.

1 1/2 cups frozen raspberries

1 banana

Ginkgo biloba (see label for recommended dosage)

Calories	197	Magnesium	66 mg
Calories from fat	14	Potassium	732 mg
Total fat	2 g	Niacin	2 mg
Carbohydrates	48 g	Vitamin B6	1 mg
Protein	3 g	Folic acid	70 mcg
Fiber	15 g	Vitamin C	57 mg

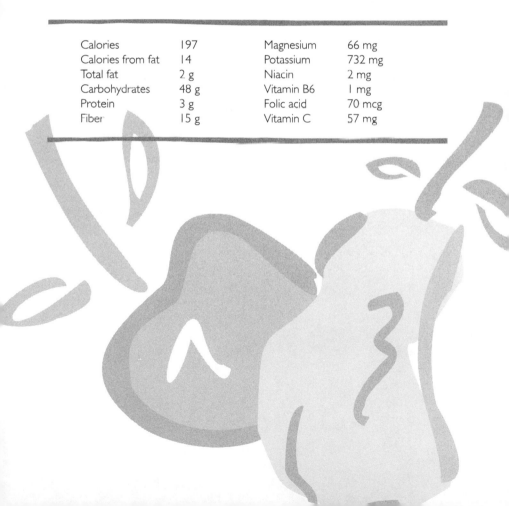

Spotted Peaches

The peaches add beta carotene and the kiwifruits add vitamin C. Both of these nutrients were shown to increase cognitive function.

1 cup drained canned peaches

3 kiwifruits, peeled

1/2 cup ice

Calories	247	Iron	2 mg
Calories from fat	10	Magnesium	89 mg
Total fat	1 g	Vitamin C	232 mg
Carbohydrates	63 g	Beta carotene	260 mcg
Protein	4 g	Vitamin E	6 mg
Fiber	11 g		

Crushed Melon Snap

Cantaloupe is an excellent source of beta carotene.

1 1/2 cups frozen cantaloupe pieces

1 1/2 cups watermelon pieces, seedless

1 (1-inch) piece fresh ginger root, peeled and crushed

200 mg vitamin C powder (see label for recommended dosage)

Calories	177	Magnesium	61 mg
Calories from fat	17	Niacin	2 mg
Total fat	2 g	Vitamin B6	1 mg
Carbohydrates	41 g	Vitamin C	248 mg
Protein	4 g	Beta carotene	7844 mcg
Fiber	3 g		

Berry Banana

You can vary the taste of this smoothie by trying different flavors of yogurt.

1 cup berry nonfat yogurt

1 cup mixed frozen berries

1 frozen banana, cut into pieces

1 tablespoon brewer's yeast

1 tablespoon lecithin granules

Calories	476	Iron	2 mg
Calories from fat	140	Zinc	2 mg
Total fat	16 g	Niacin	4 mg
Carbohydrates	79 g	Thiamin	1 mg
Protein	15 g	Vitamin B6	1 mg
Fiber	8 g	Folic acid	378 mcg

Strawberry Pears

Pears are a good source of boron.

2 canned pear halves, drained

1/2 cup frozen strawberries

1 cup pineapple juice

Ginseng supplement (see label for
recommended dosage)

Calories	204	Magnesium	48 mg
Calories from fat	5	Potassium	541 mg
Total fat	1 g	Vitamin B6	0.3 mg
Carbohydrates	51 g	Folic acid	72 mcg
Protein	2 g	Vitamin C	70 mg
Fiber	4 g		

11

Bone Builders

Smoothies to Prevent Osteoporosis

*B*one tissue is dynamic. It is constantly being laid down and taken up. During growth, bone is laid down at a greater rate than it is reabsorbed and bone mass increases. In adults, these two opposing processes proceed at equal rates, with 20 percent of an adult's bone calcium reabsorbed and replaced every year. As people age, however, the processes can reverse. In men over age fifty-five and in women past menopause, more bone can be reabsorbed than formed and bone density decreases, a condition called osteoporosis. Loss of estrogen, lack of exercise, and a poor diet all contribute to the formation of osteoporosis, and all three must be corrected to treat or prevent this disease.

Bone is made up of living bone cells (osteocytes) embedded in an organic protein matrix of collagen and osteocalcin. The calcium and phosphorus are present as calcium carbonate and calcium phosphate arranged together in a crystal structure called hydroxyapatite. Hydroxyapatite lends strength and hardness to the softer protein and osteocyte-containing matrix. Think of your bones as banks. During your teen and young adult years, you can build bone density to see you through the inevitable losses of later years.

The absorption of minerals is complicated, and a high intake of one mineral can reduce absorption of the others. Therefore, if you supplement one mineral, you should supplement them all.

GENERAL DIETARY RECOMMENDATIONS

Increase your intake of the omega-3 fatty acids. Bones grow in response to the actions of muscles. When you use your muscles, they send chemical signals to your bones that tell the bones how to form or reform. Omega-3 fatty acids are found in large quantities in fish, soybean oil, and canola oil.

Watch caffeine intake. Green tea, black tea, coffee, cocoa, chocolate, and many sodas and colas contain caffeine. Too much caffeine can dramatically increase urinary and fecal calcium loss. More than three cups of coffee a day was shown to increase the risk of hip fractures.

Do not abuse alcohol. One serving of alcohol per day will increase bone density, while heavy drinking will decrease it.

If you have a high-salt diet, reduce your intake. Salt may increase the rate of bone reabsorption and the loss of calcium in the urine.

Eat less red meat and more vegetables. Vegetarians have a lower incidence of osteoporosis than do nonvegetarians. Some researchers think that the phosphates present in red meat increase the loss of calcium in the urine.

Substitute dairy milk or soy milk for soft drinks. Soft drinks contain phosphates, which some researchers think increases the loss of calcium in the urine.

SMOOTHIE INGREDIENTS TO REDUCE OSTEOPOROSIS

Anthocyanins and Proanthocyanidins

These antioxidant flavonoids may help to stabilize the collagen matrix of bone. Anthocyanins and proanthocyanidins are found in blueberries, blackberries, cherries, raspberries, and loganberries. Add these fruits, fresh, frozen, or dried, to your smoothie.

Boron

This trace mineral interacts with calcium, magnesium, and phosphorus in bone metabolism. Boron increases the blood levels of estrogen, the female hormone involved with bone health, and aids in the conversion of vitamin D into its active form. In a study of postmenopausal women, boron supplementation decreased the urinary excretion of calcium and magnesium in women with low magnesium intakes. You can increase the boron content of your smoothies by adding apples, pears, peaches, grapes, and peanut butter.

Calcium

This mineral is the largest single component of bone. Milk, yogurt, fortified soy milk, and orange juice are sources of calcium that can be added to smoothies. A powered or liquid calcium supplement can also be added to drinks. Only about 500 mg of calcium can be absorbed at any one time, so don't rely on one supplement to supply all of your calcium needs. If you take one mineral, supplement the others to avoid deficiencies. Magnesium, calcium, and zinc all compete with each other for absorption.

Sources of Calcium for Smoothies

I cup skim milk	300 mg calcium
I/2 cup tofu set with calcium	258 mg calcium
I cup nonfat yogurt	250 mg calcium
I cup fortified orange juice	240 mg calcium
I cup cottage cheese	138 mg calcium

Fat

When fat is present in the digestive tract, it slows the movement of the stomach's content, providing more time for mineral absorption. You can add fat to your smoothie by using whole soy milk or by adding a few slices of avocado or a teaspoon of flaxseed or MCT oil.

Magnesium

This mineral is deficient in many women with osteoporosis. A high intake of calcium and vitamin D decreases the absorption of magnesium. Magnesium is available as a liquid or powder in health food stores. Or, you can add bananas, blueberries, carrot juice, cherries, dates, grapefruits, oranges, tomato juice, and raspberries to increase the magnesium content of your smoothie.

Peanuts

Peanuts are a source of protein, calcium, and boron, all ingredients necessary for healthy strong bones. Peanuts contain fat, which increases the amount of time a food spends in the stomach so that more minerals can be absorbed. They contain protein, which favors a higher absorption of calcium and phosphorus. Add a few tablespoons of peanut butter to smoothies. Choose a peanut butter that has no added hydrogenated fat or salt. Or just add shelled, unsalted peanuts to the blender for a chunkier texture.

The National Academy of Science's Institute of Medicine has released new guidelines concerning the daily intake of calcium. The guidelines recommend the following: Adolescents should have a daily intake of 1,300 mg of calcium, persons between the ages of nineteen and thirty should take in 1,000 mg, and persons over the age of fifty should take in 1,200 mg.

Soy

The isoflavonoids found in soy protein isolates, soy milk, and tofu are rich in antioxidants and phytoestrogens that may increase bone density. Soy foods also contain calcium and omega-3 fatty acids—substances needed for bone growth. Fortified soy milk is also a source of vitamin D.

Vitamin D

The sunshine vitamin is really a hormone responsible for mineral balance, and in the absence of vitamin D less than 10 percent of dietary calcium may be absorbed. Supplemental amounts of vitamin D may reduce the risk of hip fractures. Research suggests that women who take more than the recommended daily allowance (RDA) for vitamin D, along with calcium, maintain or increase bone mass instead of lose it. As you get older, your body is less efficient at manufacturing vitamin D from sunlight. It stimulates intestinal absorption of calcium and phosphorus, works with parathyroid hormone to mobilize calcium from bone, and stimulates the reabsorption of calcium from the kidneys. Soy milk, dairy milk, and yogurt are all fortified with vitamin D and make great additions to smoothies.

Vitamin K

This fat-soluble vitamin activates at least three proteins involved in bone formation. One of them, osteocalcin, needs to be saturated with chemical structures known as carboxyl groups. Vitamin K is necessary for the attachment of these groups. We may need more vitamin K than the current recommendations suggest to maintain dense, strong bones. Epidemiological evidence shows that a decrease in vitamin K is associated with an increased risk of fractures and osteoporosis. Chlorophyll and green tea extract (but not the brew) are sources of vitamin K that you can add to smoothies.

Zinc

Zinc is necessary for bone growth, and research suggests that diets deficient in this mineral may slow adolescent bone growth, which will increase the risk of developing osteoporosis later in life. A high intake of supplemental calcium can cause a zinc deficiency. Pumpkin seed butter is a rich source of vegetarian zinc that can be added to smoothies. Wheat germ, oatmeal, and soybeans also contain zinc in smaller quantities.

Green Bone Builder

The vitamin K in chlorophyll activates at least three proteins involved in bone formation.

1 cup nonfat milk

1 cup raspberries

1 frozen banana, cut into pieces

1 tablespoon brewer's yeast

1 tablespoon chlorophyll powder

Calories	277	Iron	3 mg
Calories from fat	16	Zinc	2 mg
Total fat	2 g	Niacin	5 mg
Carbohydrates	56 g	Vitamin B6	1 mg
Protein	14 g	Folic acid	380 mcg
Fiber	11 g		

You're Soy Strong!

Tofu is an good source of the calcium and protein needed for strong bones.

1 cup boysenberry nonfat yogurt

1/2 cup silken tofu

1 cup frozen blueberries, boysenberries, or raspberries (or other berries)

Calories	398	Calcium	489 mg
Calories from fat	74	Iron	3 mg
Total fat	8 g	Potassium	581 mg
Carbohydrates	66 g	Zinc	2 mg
Protein	19 g	Riboflavin	0.5 mg
Fiber	4 g		

The Golden One

Ground sesame seeds, or tahini, and dates are sources of calcium, magnesium, and fiber.

1 cup nonfat yogurt

1/2 cup nonfat milk

1/4 cup dates, pitted and chopped

1 frozen banana, cut into pieces

3 tablespoons tahini (ground sesame seeds)

Powdered calcium/magnesium supplement
   (see label for recommended dosage)

Calories	682	Calcium	814 mg
Calories from fat	249	Iron	5 mg
Total fat	28 g	Magnesium	150 mg
Carbohydrates	92 g	Potassium	1695 mg
Protein	27 g	Zinc	5 mg
Fiber	9 g	Niacin	4 mg

Bouncing Lizbet

Magnesium is deficient in many women with osteoporosis. The fruits in this recipe are all sources of this important mineral.

1 cup nonfat milk

1/2 cup frozen blueberries

1/2 cup frozen cherries

1 banana

Calories	284	Calcium	324 mg
Calories from fat	18	Magnesium	73 mg
Total fat	2 g	Riboflavin	1 mg
Carbohydrates	61 g	Vitamin B6	1 mg
Protein	11 g	Vitamin A	182 mcg
Fiber	6 g		

Girl Power

This smoothie is rich in the isoflavonoids, vitamin D, and calcium, which prevent osteoporosis.

1 cup fortified soy milk

1 frozen banana, cut into pieces

3 to 4 dates, pitted and chopped

1 tablespoon flaxseed powder

Calcium/magnesium supplement (see label for recommended dosage)

200 to 300 mg vitamin C powder (see label for recommended dosage)

Calories	341	Iron	6 mg
Calories from fat	75	Magnesium	113 mg
Total fat	8 g	Vitamin B6	1 mg
Carbohydrates	59 g	Vitamin C	210 mg
Protein	13 g	Vitamin E	8 mg
Fiber	9 g		

Gingered Cherry Cream

Soy foods contain calcium and omega-3 fatty acids, substances needed for bone growth.

1 cup cherry nonfat yogurt

1/2 cup silken tofu

1 cup frozen cherries

1 (1-inch) piece fresh ginger root, peeled and crushed

Calories	436	Calcium	506 mg
Calories from fat	83	Iron	3 mg
Total fat	9 g	Potassium	864 mg
Carbohydrates	72 g	Riboflavin	1 mg
Protein	20 g	Vitamin B12	1 mcg
Fiber	4 g		

Orange Coconut Cooler

This smoothie is light and creamy but rich in flavor.

1 cup calcium-fortified orange juice

1 apple, cored, peeled, and sliced

1 orange, peeled and seeded

2 tablespoons lowfat coconut milk

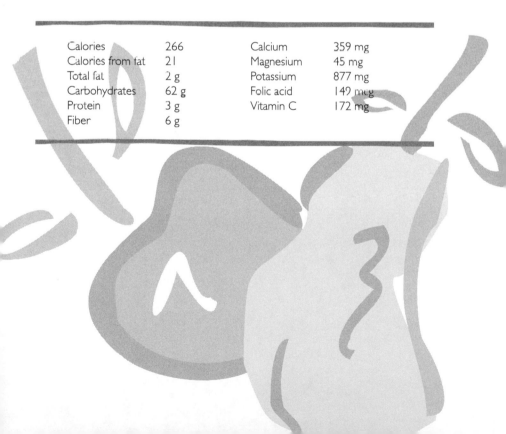

Calories	266	Calcium	359 mg
Calories from fat	21	Magnesium	45 mg
Total fat	2 g	Potassium	877 mg
Carbohydrates	62 g	Folic acid	149 mcg
Protein	3 g	Vitamin C	172 mg
Fiber	6 g		

Berry Crush

The anthocyanins and proanthocyanidins found in berries help to stabilize the collagen matrix of bone.

1/2 cup orange juice

1 orange, peeled, seeded, and sliced

1 cup frozen raspberries

1 cup frozen blueberries

Calories	204	Potassium	553 mg
Calories from fat	13	Niacin	2 mg
Total fat	1 g	Folic acid	81 mcg
Carbohydrates	50 g	Vitamin C	120 mg
Protein	3 g	Vitamin E	2 mg
Fiber	15 g		

Tropical Shake

Fortified soy milk contains the vitamin D, calcium, and magnesium found in dairy milk plus the isoflavones that prevent bone thinning.

1 cup fortified nonfat soy milk

1 cup pineapple juice

1 frozen banana, cut into pieces

2 tablespoons lowfat coconut milk

1 tablespoon shredded coconut

Calories	368	Calcium	252 mg
Calories from fat	52	Iron	3 mg
Total fat	6 g	Magnesium	76 mg
Carbohydrates	78 g	Potassium	835 mg
Protein	5 g	Vitamin B6	1 mg
Fiber	4 g		

Java Shake

Here's coffee with a shake.

10 ounces fortified milk or soy milk

1 frozen banana, cut into pieces

1 to 2 tablespoons instant coffee powder

Calories	225	Calcium	393 mg
Calories from fat	10	Magnesium	86 mg
Total fat	1 g	Riboflavin	1 mg
Carbohydrates	44 g	Niacin	2 mg
Protein	12 g	Vitamin B6	1 mg
Fiber	3 g		

Strawberry Cheesecake

The calcium found in the fortified orange juice and cottage cheese helps to build strong bones.

1 1/2 cups strawberries

1 cup nonfat cottage cheese

1/2 cup fortified orange juice

Calories	264	Calcium	302 mg
Calories from fat	8	Iron	1 mg
Total fat	1 g	Potassium	608 mg
Carbohydrates	37 g	Folic acid	94 mcg
Protein	30 g	Vitamin C	175 mg
Fiber	5 g		

Chocolate Pears

In this smoothie, the delicate taste of pears is combined with the smooth taste of chocolate.

1 cup fortified cocoa soy milk

4 canned pear halves, drained

2 tablespoons chocolate sauce

Calories	337	Fiber	7 g
Calories from fat	39	Iron	3 mg
Total fat	4 g	Potassium	521 mg
Carbohydrates	71 g	Niacin	1 mg
Protein	8 g	Folic acid	40 mcg

Vanilla and Blueberries

Blueberries contain the flavonoid pigment anthocyanin, which together with ascorbic acid (vitamin C) supports the growth of collagen and the protein in bone tissue.

1 cup vanilla nonfat yogurt

1 1/2 cups frozen blueberries

1 teaspoon pure vanilla extract

Calories	322	Calcium	465 mg
Calories from fat	11	Magnesium	54 mg
Total fat	1 g	Zinc	2 mg
Carbohydrates	64 g	Riboflavin	1 mg
Protein	15 g	Vitamin B12	1 mcg
Fiber	6 g		

Mango Shake

Enjoy this thick, sweet shake rich in beta carotene, boron, calcium, and magnesium.

1 1/2 cups mango slices

1 frozen banana, cut into pieces

1 cup nonfat milk

Calcium/magnesium supplement (see label for recommended dosage)

Calories	353	Vitamin B6	1 mg
Calories from fat	15	Vitamin C	82 mg
Total fat	2 g	Vitamin A	1126 mcg
Carbohydrates	81 g	Beta carotene	773 mcg
Protein	11 g	Vitamin E	3 mg
Fiber	7 g		

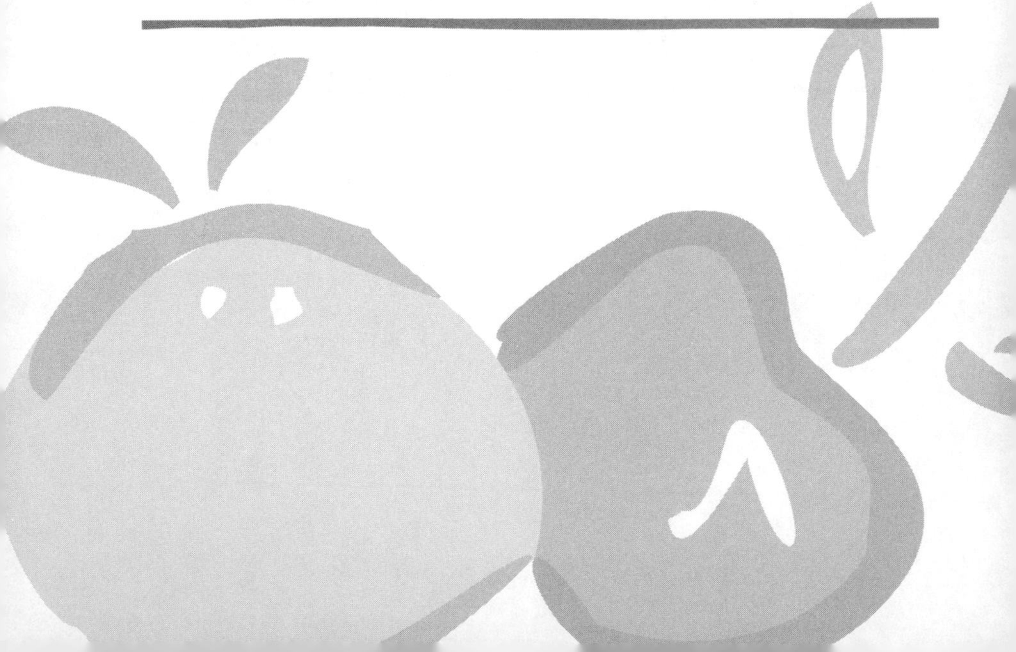

12

Healing Tonics and Restoratives

Smoothies That Heal

*P*lant foods are brimming full of phytochemicals that can be used to treat a wide variety of minor ailments and illnesses. No food or herb should substitute for qualified medical care or advice, but in many instances minor aches and pains can be relieved by the many remedies present in nature's medicine cabinet.

SMOOTHIE INGREDIENTS FOR TONICS AND RESTORATIVES

Antioxidants

Antioxidants help to support the immune system during colds and the flu. They may help to shorten the duration of a cold. You can find antioxidant supplements to add to smoothies at your health food store in liquid and powder form. All yellow, orange, and red fruits and vegetables are sources of antioxidants.

Bananas

Bananas have a soothing effect on upset stomachs and reduce stomach acidity. Add either frozen or fresh bananas to your smoothie when your stomach is on the queasy side.

Bran

Bran (wheat, rice, and oat) are concentrated sources of fiber that will increase the bulk and frequency of bowel movements by attracting water into the feces. Wheat bran holds three times its weight in water, and rice bran may hold even more. Soluble bran such as oat bran may also be effective. Start with one teaspoon and gradually work up to one tablespoon.

Brewer's Yeast

Brewer's yeast is the best source of the B-complex vitamins. They are necessary for the release of energy and for the production of neuro-transmitters.

Cinnamon, Apple Pie Spice, Cloves, and Peanut Butter

Cinnamon, apple pie spice, cloves, and peanut butter contain an insulin-tolerance factor that helps the body to utilize insulin more efficiently.

Coffee

Coffee is a source of caffeine, a natural stimulant. In some people it has a laxative action that works within minutes. Add one tablespoon of in-stant coffee to your smoothie.

Cranberries

The most common bacteria that causes urinary tract infection is *Escherichia coli*. This bacteria produces chemicals that allow it to stick to the walls of the bladder. Cranberry juice contains two substances that inhibit the ability of bacteria to adhere to surfaces: fructose and an as yet unidentified polymeric compound.

Ginger

Ginger root is a source of the trace mineral zinc. It works as a blood thinner, preventing the formation of dangerous blood clots, and is an effective remedy for the prevention of motion sickness and nausea of pregnancy. Some studies have shown that ginger can prevent migraine headaches. It also has use as a natural inflammatory agent. You can add fresh peeled ginger root or ginger root powder to smoothies.

Magnesium/Calcium/Potassium

These minerals are involved in muscle and nerve contraction. They are of use whenever muscles cramp or experience fatigue. Fruits and vegetables rich in minerals are linked with lower blood pressure levels.

Nutmeg

This spice reduces peristalsis (natural contractions of the colon). Add it to smoothies when diarrhea is a problem. Add a liberal sprinkle of fresh-ground nutmeg to your smoothie.

Papaya

Papaya is a tropical fruit that contains the protein-digesting enzyme papain. Papain is used to improve digestion and is also a natural anti-inflammatory agent.

Peppermint

Peppermint stimulates bile flow and appetite and aids in digestion. It acts as a carminative, relaxing the smooth muscle of the digestive tract, and is often recommended for "gas" pain. Add a few drops of peppermint oil or a few peppermint leaves to your smoothie.

Pineapple

This fruit is a source of bromelain, an enzyme that digests protein. Bromelain is a natural anti-inflammatory agent and helps dissolve blood clots.

Prunes

Prunes are famous for their laxative action. They are also rich in natural aspirin and a good source of iron. Prunes are full of fiber. Add either whole pitted prunes or prune juice to your smoothie. Pitted prunes now come in a variety of flavors such as lemon and orange.

Psyllium Seed

Psyllium seed contains a water-absorbing substance called mucilage. The mucilage in psyllium seed can swell to ten times its original size in the presence of water. This increases the bulk of feces, alleviating constipation. The water-absorbing properties of psyllium seed also alleviates diarrhea. This makes psyllium seed powder a valuable food in the treatment of irritable bowel syndrome. Psyllium seed powder is also used to treat high cholesterol and in animal studies has been shown to reduce blood sugar. Add one teaspoon of ground psyllium seed to your smoothie and gradually work up to one tablespoon.

Pumpkin Seeds

Pumpkin seeds contain alanine, glutamic acid, and glycine, the amino acids used to treat prostate enlargement. Ground pumpkin seeds (pumpkin seed butter) can be added to smoothies to increase their fat content.

Resveratrol

This substance found in mulberries, peanuts, and in the skin of red and white grapes may be a potent cancer-preventing agent. Researchers have found that resveratrol inhibits all three major stages of carcinogenesis: initiation, promotion, and progression. Wine, purple grape juice, and peanut butter are sources of resveratrol that can be added to smoothies.

Foods High in Salicylates (A Natural Form of Aspirin)

Almonds	Loganberries
Apricots	Mint
Blackberries	Nutmeg
Blueberries	Oranges
Boysenberries	Peanuts
Cantaloupes	Pineapples
Cherries	Plums
Cranberries	Prunes
Currants	Raisins
Dates	Raspberries
Ginger root	Strawberries
Grapes (sultana)	Tomato paste
Guavas	Vanilla
Licorice	

Vitamin C

This antioxidant vitamin acts as a natural antihistamine. Powdered ascorbic acid (vitamin C) can be added to smoothies.

Yogurt

Yogurt is a cultured milk product that is a natural source of friendly bacteria and a natural antibiotic. Choose a brand that is low in fat and that contains live cultures of bacteria (it will be stated on the container, so always look for it).

Ginger Jolt

This is a good smoothie for a queasy tummy. Drink it slowly.

1 apple, cored, peeled, and sliced

1 lemon, peeled and seeded

1/2 cup filtered water

1/2 cup ice

1 (2-inch) piece fresh ginger root, peeled
and crushed

Calories	120	Protein	2 g
Calories from fat	8	Fiber	5 g
Total fat	1 g	Magnesium	30 mg
Carbohydrates	30 g	Potassium	400 mg

Tummy Soother

The banana in this smoothie soothes the irritated stomach, while the ginger prevents nausea.

1/2 frozen banana, cut into pieces

1 cup nonfat milk

1/2 to 1 capsule ginger root powder

Calories	140	Calcium	306 mg
Calories from fat	6	Potassium	638 mg
Total fat	1 g	Riboflavin	0.4 mg
Carbohydrates	26 g	Vitamin B12	1 mcg
Protein	9 g	Vitamin B6	0.4 mg
Fiber	1 g		

Hot Redhead with a Secret

The secret in this veggie smoothie is the garlic. Garlic and onions contain dozens of medicinal compounds.

1 cup tomato juice

1/2 teaspoon chopped jalapeño pepper

1/4 teaspoon cayenne

1/4 cup chopped onion

1/2 cup chopped parsley

2 cloves garlic, peeled

Calories	79	Vitamin B6	0.4 mg
Calories from fat	5	Folic acid	97 mcg
Total fat	1 g	Vitamin C	87 mg
Carbohydrates	18 g	Vitamin A	294 mcg
Protein	4 g	Beta carotene	3797 mcg
Fiber	3 g	Vitamin E	3 mg
Niacin	2 mg		

Orange Buzz

This smoothie combines propolis and honey, two products of bees with immune-enhancing properties.

1/2 cup fresh orange juice

1/2 cup fresh carrot juice

1/2 cup frozen peach, apricot, or mango slices

1/2 lemon, peeled and seeded

1 teaspoon honey

1 tablespoon propolis

Calories	171	Niacin	2 mg
Calories from fat	5	Vitamin B6	0.4 mg
Total fat	1 g	Folic acid	49 mcg
Carbohydrates	42 g	Vitamin C	93 mg
Protein	3 g	Beta carotene	12185 mcg
Fiber	4 g		

Creamy Cranberry

This smoothie contains blueberries and cranberries, which aid in the prevention of bladder infections.

1 cup frozen blueberries

1/4 cup frozen whole cranberries

1/2 cup vanilla nonfat yogurt

1/2 cup cranberry juice cocktail

Calories	260		Calcium	240 mg
Calories from fat	8		Potassium	466 mg
Total fat	1 g		Riboflavin	0.4 mg
Carbohydrates	59 g		Vitamin B12	1 mcg
Protein	8 g		Vitamin C	77 mg
Fiber	5 g			

Strawberry-Orange Shake

Here's a smooth way to get extra vitamin C and bioflavonoids, to ward off those summer colds.

1 cup orange juice

1 cup frozen strawberries

1 frozen banana, cut into pieces

200 mg vitamin C powder

Liquid herbal extract of choice, optional

Calories	342	Iron	4 mg
Calories from fat	59	Zinc	2 mg
Total fat	7 g	Vitamin B6	1 mg
Carbohydrates	50 g	Folic acid	194 mcg
Protein	25 g	Vitamin C	97 mg
Fiber	6 g		

Nutty Raspberries

Raspberries and prunes are rich in salicylates, a form of natural aspirin. They may also help prevent the free radical damage that initiates heart disease.

1 cup frozen raspberries

1/4 cup prune puree

1/4 cup nonfat milk or soy milk

2 tablespoons almond butter or peanut butter

Calories	330	Iron	2 mg
Calories from fat	178	Magnesium	130 mg
Total fat	20 g	Zinc	2 mg
Carbohydrates	36 g	Niacin	2 mg
Protein	9 g	Vitamin E	7 mg
Fiber	10 g		

Yogurt Cooler

Make sure that the yogurt you buy contains live bacterial cultures. Look for this information on the label. Yogurt with live cultures has antibacterial and antifungal properties and is especially useful for female infections.

1 1/2 cups plain nonfat yogurt
1 cup blackberries
1/2 cup fresh pineapple juice

Calories	335	Calcium	745 mg
Calories from fat	12	Potassium	1318 mg
Total fat	1 g	Zinc	4 mg
Carbohydrates	62 g	Riboflavin	1 mg
Protein	21 g	Folic acid	120 mcg
Fiber	8 g		

Tropical Treatment

The sweetness of this drink will help to hide the taste of any bitter herbal extract.

1 cup fresh or frozen mango pieces

1/2 cup guava nectar

1/2 frozen banana, cut into pieces

1 teaspoon fresh lime juice

1 teaspoon herbal extract, optional

Calories	223	Vitamin B6	0.5 mg
Calories from fat	9	Vitamin C	76 mg
Total fat	1 g	Vitamin A	576 mcg
Carbohydrates	57 g	Potassium	496 mg
Protein	2 g	Beta carotene	571 mcg
Fiber	4 g		

Banana Soother

This is a good smoothie for an upset stomach. Mint leaves reduce contractions of the gastrointestinal tract muscle, while banana soothes the irritation of the stomach lining.

1 cup rice milk

1 frozen banana, cut into pieces

4 to 5 mint leaves

Calories	160	Fiber	3 g
Calories from fat	9	Magnesium	44 mg
Total fat	1 g	Potassium	494 mg
Carbohydrates	40 g	Vitamin B6	0.7 mg
Protein	55 g		

Ginger Warmer

Ginger and pineapple contain natural anti-inflammatory agents that can help to reduce the pain and stiffness of arthritis.

1 cup apple juice

1 cup fresh pineapple pieces

1 frozen banana, cut into pieces

1 (1-inch) piece fresh ginger root, peeled and crushed

Calories	315	Magnesium	69 mg
Calories from fat	18	Potassium	1009 mg
Total fat	2 g	Thiamin	0.3 mg
Carbohydrates	78 g	Vitamin B6	0.9 mg
Protein	2 g	Vitamin C	38 mg
Fiber	5 g		

Blueberry Berry

All of the ingredients in this smoothie work to normalize overactive colon contractions. Soak the dried blueberries in the rice milk for a few minutes before making the smoothie.

1 cup frozen blueberries

1 cup rice milk

1/2 cup dried blueberries, presoaked

1 teaspoon psyllium seed powder

1 teaspoon ground nutmeg

Calories	445	Protein	57 g
Calories from fat	18	Fiber	20 g
Total fat	2 g	Iron	4 mg
Carbohydrates	108 g	Vitamin E	2 mg

Purple Papaya

This drink is filled with natural anti-inflammatory agents and antioxidants. They will help to prevent and treat heart disease, cancer, and hypertension.

1 cup purple grape juice

1 cup fresh or frozen papaya slices

Calories	182	Fiber	3 g
Calories from fat	0	Folic acid	56 mcg
Total fat	0 g	Vitamin C	146 mg
Carbohydrates	46 g	Vitamin A	284 mcg
Protein	1 g	Vitamin E	2 mg

Apricots and Apples

This smoothie is a good choice for those with high cholesterol. Both the psyllium seed and the pectin found in the apples reduce blood cholesterol levels.

1 cup drained canned apricots

1 apple, cored, peeled, and sliced

1 cup apple juice

Calories	350	Fiber	8 g
Calories from fat	9	Iron	2 mg
Total fat	1 g	Niacin	2 mg
Carbohydrates	90 g	Beta Carotene	3435 mcg
Protein	3 g	Vitamin E	3 mg

Pineapple Ginger Iced Tea

Green tea has antiviral properties, and the pineapple and ginger root reduce inflammation. Sip this tea next time you have a cold or the flu.

1 cup brewed green tea, cooled

1 cup fresh pineapple chunks

1/2 cup ice

1 (1-inch) piece fresh ginger root, peeled and crushed

Calories	94	Protein	1 g
Calories from fat	9	Fiber	2 g
Total fat	1 g	Magnesium	33 mg
Carbohydrates	23 g	Potassium	283 mg

13

Detoxifiers
Smoothies to Purify

*T*he liver is the organ responsible for detoxifying chemicals that work their way into your body: the pesticides and herbicides on produce, the hormones in meat and dairy products, the carbon monoxide in the air, and the tobacco smoke blown in your face, for example. The effect these poisons have on your body is directly related to how well your body can detoxify them.

You can help your body to process these toxins by providing it with the vitamins, minerals, and amino acids needed by the liver for the detoxification process. Soluble fiber in the intestine will help to bind excreted toxins, and insoluble fiber will promote prompt elimination.

The colonic bacteria also play a role in the detoxification process. The proper bacteria will aid in the process. Other less-desirable types will only add to the toxic burden.

GENERAL DIETARY RECOMMENDATIONS

Eat a diet rich in plant foods. Plants contain a wide variety of substances that act as detoxifiers and antioxidants.

Eat generous amount of garlic, onions, and leeks. These foods are excellent sources of sulfur compounds needed for detoxification. Wash all your produce carefully in soapy warm water, and buy organic fruits and vegetables when you can. This will decrease your exposure to pesticides used on plants.

Avoid alcohol during periods when your liver is under stress. Excess alcohol depletes your body's store of natural detoxifiers.

Drink eight to ten glasses of water of day. This helps the kidneys to eliminate toxin breakdown products.

SMOOTHIE INGREDIENTS TO DETOXIFY

Acidophilus and Bifidus Bacteria

Acidophilus and bifidus bacteria are an important tool in maintaining a healthy digestive tract. They help to keep the colon populated with healthy bacteria, thereby avoiding microbial toxins. You can add these live bacteria to your smoothies as part of dairy milk with added acidophilus or as a separate acidophilus or bifidus supplement.

Avocados

The avocado is one of the richest sources of glutathione, a potent antioxidant that can detoxify environmental pollutants. It also contains vitamin E, another antioxidant, and enough oil to ensure that this fat-soluble vitamin is absorbed.

Brewer's Yeast

The folic acid pyridoxine (vitamin B6) and vitamin B12 in brewer's yeast help to detoxify homocysteine, a protein found in the blood of some people. Homocysteine is toxic to the arterial cell wall and is associated with an increased risk of heart disease.

Chlorella

This algae is used in the detoxification of heavy metals such as cadmium, uranium, and lead. Studies in Japan have shown that chlorella increases the excretion of cadmium from victims of cadmium poisoning. In the lab rat, substances from the chlorella cell wall reduce the half-life of synthetically produced hydrocarbons such as PCBs (polychlorinated biphenyls) and the pesticide chlordecone. Powdered chlorella is available at health food stores. Add one teaspoon to your smoothies.

Glutathione

This amino acid is an important source of sulfur for the body. Sulfur-containing compounds function as detoxifying agents by combining with toxic substances, making them water soluble so that they can be excreted through the kidneys. Glutathione is a sulfur-containing compound that is found in oranges, watermelon, strawberries, avocados, and carrots.

Malic Acid

This weak acid is a powerful chelator of iron and aluminum. It is found naturally in apples and pears, or it can be purchased as a powder.

Psyllium Seed

Psyllium seeds are rich sources of a soluble fiber called mucilage. The mucilage in psyllium seed aids in colon health. It prevents constipation and binds cholesterol and toxins in the intestine. When added to water, psyllium seed powder can swell to ten times its original size. It is odorless and bland in taste but has a gritty texture that is reduced by adding it to a drink containing a frozen fruit. Start with one teaspoon of psyllium seed powder and gradually work up to one tablespoon, to avoid developing gas.

Soluble Fiber

Soluble fiber is a type of carbohydrate that resists digestion by gastrointestinal secretions. It dissolves in the watery contents of the small intestine, producing a viscous gel. Soluble fiber binds toxins in the colon. It also will decrease the chance of constipation and lower cholesterol levels. Psyllium seed powder, flaxseed powder, oat bran, and pectin are all soluble fiber sources that can be added to smoothies. Start with one teaspoon, working gradually up to one tablespoon.

HERBS TO DETOXIFY

Chinese or Korean Ginseng

Chinese or Korean ginseng (*Panax ginseng*) has been used for centuries as a whole body tonic. It is thought to enhance the ability of the Kupffer cells of the liver to filter toxins from the bloodstream.

Silymarin

This extract of the milk thistle plant is a well-documented, powerful antioxidant that prevents free radical damage to the liver and stimulates the synthesis of protein for the formation of new liver cells. It also prevents the depletion of the antioxidant glutathione, which aids in the detoxification of alcohol. Silymarin is available in liquid form to add to smoothies.

Sweet and Sour

A powerful blend of antioxidants in this smoothie protect your liver from toxin-induced free radical damage.

1 orange, peeled and seeded

1 lime, peeled and seeded

1/2 peach, pitted and peeled

1/2 nectarine, pitted and peeled

1/2 cup ice

Silymarin (see label for recommended dosage)

Calories	134	Potassium	535 mg
Calories from fat	5	Niacin	2 mg
Total fat	1 g	Folic acid	49 mcg
Carbohydrates	35 g	Vitamin C	96 mg
Protein	3 g	Vitamin A	102 mcg
Fiber	7 g		

Tropical Rush

This smoothie is a good source of both soluble and insoluble fiber. The bacterial cultures will help to re-establish healthful bacterial populations in your colon.

1 cup cantaloupe pieces

1 cup fresh or frozen pineapple chunks

1/2 orange, peeled and seeded

1/4 cup ice

Acidophilus supplement (see label for recommended dosage)

1 teaspoon psyllium seed powder

Calories	165	Potassium	820 mg
Calories from fat	11	Niacin	2 mg
Total fat	1 g	Vitamin C	75 mg
Carbohydrates	44 g	Vitamin A	534 mcg
Protein	3 g	Beta carotene	4859 mcg
Fiber	8 g		

Short Sea Freeze

This cold, creamy smoothie features chlorella, a sea algae that is used for the detoxification of heavy metals such as cadmium, uranium, and lead.

1 cup rice milk

1/2 cup flavored nonfat frozen yogurt

1 teaspoon chlorella

200 mg vitamin C powder

Calories	194	Fiber	0 g
Calories from fat	3	Potassium	210 mg
Total fat	0 g	Vitamin B12	1 mcg
Carbohydrates	36 g	Vitamin C	200 mg
Protein	68 g		

Short Sea Goddess

Acidophilus and bifidus bacteria are important tools in maintaining a healthy digestive tract. They help to replenish the flora of the colon when it has been depleted by stress or antibiotics.

1 cup nonfat milk

1/2 cup flavored nonfat frozen yogurt

2 tablespoons plain or flavored nonfat yogurt

1 teaspoon chlorella

Acidophilus supplement (see label for recommended dosage)

1/2 teaspoon pure vanilla extract

Calories	251	Calcium	441 mg
Calories from fat	5	Potassium	674 mg
Total fat	1 g	Zinc	2 mg
Carbohydrates	37 g	Riboflavin	1 mg
Protein	24 g	Vitamin B12	2 mcg
Fiber	0 g		

Orange High

This smoothie is a good source of glutathione, a powerful anti-oxidant, and malic acid, a potent chelator of heavy minerals.

1 orange, peeled and seeded

1 cup applesauce

1/2 cup ice

Acidophilus supplement (see label for recommended dosage)

1 teaspoon psyllium seed powder

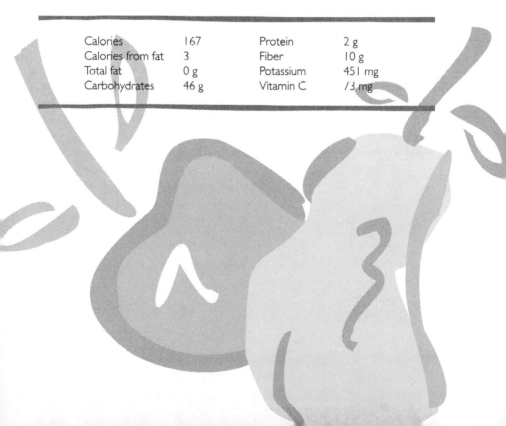

Calories	167	Protein	2 g
Calories from fat	3	Fiber	10 g
Total fat	0 g	Potassium	451 mg
Carbohydrates	46 g	Vitamin C	73 mg

Purple Shake

The banana in this drink supplies vitamin B6, the brewer's yeast contributes vitamin B12, and the orange juice adds folic acid. All of these vitamins are necessary for the detoxification of homo-cysteine, a protein that is toxic to the cell walls of arteries.

1 cup purple grape juice

1/2 cup frozen blueberries

1/2 cup orange juice

1 frozen banana, cut into pieces

1 tablespoon brewer's yeast

Calories	369	Iron	3 mg
Calories from fat	12	Magnesium	75 mg
Total fat	1 g	Riboflavin	1 mg
Carbohydrates	84 g	Niacin	5 mg
Protein	10 g	Folic acid	352 mcg
Fiber	5 g		

Sea Tea

Here's a summer alternative to hot tea or coffee. This smoothie contains a small amount of caffeine to boost your energy levels and mental awareness.

1 cup brewed green or black tea, cooled

1 cup frozen watermelon pieces, seedless

2 to 3 ice cubes

1 teaspoon algae

Calories	70	Fiber	1 g
Calories from fat	10	Iron	2 mg
Total fat	1 g	Potassium	352 mg
Carbohydrates	14 g	Niacin	1 mg
Protein	4 g	Beta carotene	388 mcg

Apricot Shake

The wheat germ provides insoluble fiber and the oat bran supplies soluble fiber, both of which aid the colon in excreting toxins.

1 1/2 cups drained canned apricots

1 frozen banana, cut into pieces

1/2 cup soy milk

1 tablespoon oat bran

1 tablespoon wheat germ

Calories	314	Iron	3 mg
Calories from fat	37	Magnesium	112 mg
Total fat	4 g	Vitamin B6	1 mg
Carbohydrates	70 g	Beta carotene	2697 mcg
Protein	9 g	Vitamin E	4 mg
Fiber	11 g		

Watermelon Cooler

This smoothie is rich in glutathione, which is part of the powerful liver enzyme glutathione peroxidase.

1 cup watermelon pieces, seedless

1/2 cup frozen strawberries

1 orange, peeled and seeded

Calories	136	Potassium	551 mg
Calories from fat	10	Vitamin B6	0.4 mg
Total fat	1 g	Folic acid	56 mcg
Carbohydrates	32 g	Vitamin C	128 mg
Protein	3 g	Beta carotene	433 mcg
Fiber	6 g		

Peachy Citrus Crush

Add your favorite ginseng extract to this smoothie.

1 cup drained canned peaches

1/2 cup ice

1 orange, peeled and seeded

1/2 lemon, peeled and seeded

Liquid ginseng extract (see label for
  recommended dosage)

Calories	180	Niacin	2 mg
Calories from fat	3	Vitamin C	94 mg
Total fat	0 g	Vitamin A	121 mcg
Carbohydrates	47 g	Beta carotene	213 mcg
Protein	3 g	Vitamin E	4 mg
Fiber	7 g		

Cinnamon Pears

Fiber is often called "nature's broom" because of its ability to clean out the colon. Each pear in this smoothie contains 5 grams of fiber.

4 canned pear halves, drained

1/2 cup orange juice

1 teaspoon ground cinnamon

Calories	214	Iron	2 mg
Calories from fat	3	Potassium	544 mg
Total fat	0 g	Folic acid	59 mcg
Carbohydrates	55 g	Vitamin C	54 mg
Protein	2 g	Vitamin E	2 mg
Fiber	6 g		

Pear-Apple Snap

Pears and apples contain malic acid, a heavy metal chelator.

4 canned pear halves, drained

1/2 apple, peeled, cored, and sliced

1/2 cup apple juice

1 teaspoon psyllium seed powder

1 (2-inch) piece fresh ginger, peeled and crushed

Calories	277	Iron	2 mg
Calories from fat	9	Magnesium	44 mg
Total fat	1 g	Potassium	720 mg
Carbohydrates	73 g	Niacin	1 mg
Protein	2 g	Vitamin E	2 mg
Fiber	10 g		

14

Balancers

Smoothies for Women

*B*ecause women carry and bear the young, nature has given them an often complicated and not well understood hormonal system. Imbalances in this system cause problems before menses (premenstrual syndrome, or PMS), during menses (cramps, heavy bleeding), during pregnancy (nausea), in later life (perimenopause), and after the stop of menses (menopausal symptoms). Luckily, it is rare that a woman has problems at every stage of life.

Women who continue to have problems at any stage of life should see their gynecologist for guidance.

GENERAL DIETARY RECOMMENDATIONS

After menopause, it is more important for women to watch their intake of saturated fat. To reduce saturated fats, eliminate butter and butterfat from your diet. Consume only skim milk and non-fat dairy products.

Eat generous amounts of cruciferous vegetables, such as broccoli, kale, and cauliflower. These vegetables contain a substance that aids in the detoxification of estrogen, decreasing the chances that this hormone can promote breast cancer.

Substitute soy nuts for high-fat snacks. Two tablespoons of roasted soy nuts contain about 30 mg of estrogen-replacing isoflavones.

Watch your intake of caffeine. For some women, as little as one cup a day of a caffeine-containing beverage can cause PMS symptoms.

If you suffer from PMS, eat a diet rich in carbohydrates. Time meals and snacks so that you do not go more than three hours on an empty stomach. Start each meal with a small amount of a starchy carbohydrate.

SMOOTHIE INGREDIENTS FOR WOMEN

Brewer's Yeast

Brewer's yeast is an excellent source of all the B-complex vitamins. A tablespoon of brewer's yeast will help replenish the B vitamins lost from stress, alcohol abuse, and the use of birth control pills and alcohol.

Calcium

Calcium is involved in nerve transmission and muscle contraction. Studies have shown that increasing levels of calcium can prevent mood changes during the week prior to menstruation. Cramps and headaches were also reduced during menstruation. Calcium can be used to control the incidence of leg cramps in pregnant women, possibly by decreasing nerve irritability. Yogurt, dairy milk, fortified soy milk, cottage cheese, and tofu are all sources of calcium that can be used in smoothies. Liquid or powdered calcium supplement can be added.

Flaxseed Powder

Flaxseed powder (also called ground flaxseed) is a wonderful source of fiber and isoflavones.

Iron

Iron carries oxygen in the blood and is a nutrient often found to be deficient in women. Vitamin C helps the body absorb iron more efficiently. In smoothies, combine soy milk or tofu with vitamin C–containing ingredients to create an iron-rich elixir. Iron can be added to smoothies as part of a protein or multivitamin/mineral supplement. Prunes, raisins, tofu, pumpkin seeds, and wheat germ will increase the iron content of smoothies. Citrus fruits, strawberries, papaya, and mangoes are good sources of vitamin C.

Magnesium

Brain levels of this mineral have been found to be low in migraine sufferers. Menstrual migraine sufferers have an intracellular magnesium deficiency, and oral magnesium supplementation improves both migraine and other premenstrual complaints. Magnesium is available as a liquid in health food stores. Or you can add bananas, blueberries, carrot juice, cherries, dates, grapefruits, oranges, tomato juice, and raspberries to increase the magnesium content of your smoothies.

Manganese

A deficiency in this mineral can be the cause of heavy menstrual periods. Add tea, pineapple, and strawberries to your smoothie to increase manganese levels.

Soy Milk and Tofu

These soy foods are rich in phytoestrogens and can cool the hot flashes of menopause by acting as natural estrogen replacement therapy. A study presented at a recent American Heart Association meeting reported that women who had hot flashes at least once a day were given soy powder containing 34 mg of isoflavones. During six weeks on soy, the women's hot flashes became significantly less intense. An equivalent amount of isoflavones can also be found in one-half cup of tofu or one and a half cups of soy milk. Other sources of phytoestrogens for smoothies include peanut butter, almonds, oranges, flaxseed powder or oil, and sunflower seeds.

Vitamins K, C, and B6

Low pyridoxine (vitamin B6) levels are common among pregnant women and may be a contributing factor to morning sickness. Vitamin C and vitamin K taken together have shown dramatic clinical effects in halting morning sickness.

HERBS FOR WOMEN

Ginseng

Ginseng's healing properties are believed to be due to a family of chemicals called ginsenosides. In postmenopausal women, ginsenosides acted like estrogen on the cells lining the vagina, preventing the cells from atrophying.

Licorice

This pleasant-tasting herb possesses estrogenic activity and is used to decrease the symptoms of menopause and PMS. Look for a liquid licorice root extract in health food stores.

Peppermint

The menthol found in the mint leaf is an antispasmodic that can be used to soothe the lining of the digestive tract and decrease menstrual cramps.

Licorice Cream

The ingredients in this smoothie highlight the taste of the licorice supplement.

1 cup fortified vanilla soy milk

1/2 cup vanilla lowfat frozen yogurt

1/2 cup silken tofu

500 mg calcium liquid or powder

Licorice root extract (see label for
  recommended dosage)

Calories	317	Fiber	2 g
Calories from fat	80	Calcium	736 mg
Total fat	9 g	Iron	4 mg
Carbohydrates	40 g	Potassium	210 mg
Protein	17 g		

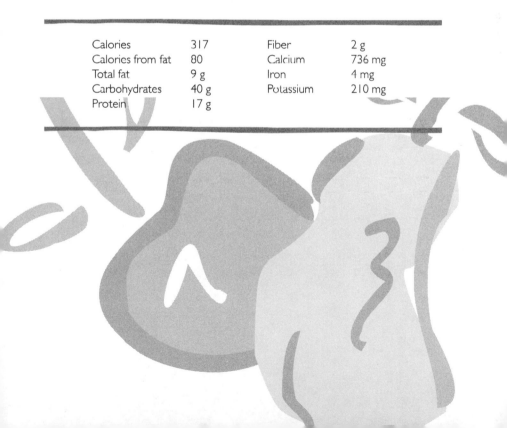

Berry Cream

The soy protein in this drink contains isoflavones that relieve menopausal symptoms.

1 cup fortified soy milk

1/2 cup silken tofu

1/2 cup raspberry nonfat frozen yogurt

1/2 cup frozen berries

1/2 teaspoon acidophilus powder

Calories	379	Calcium	435 mg
Calories from fat	98	Iron	5 mg
Total fat	11 g	Magnesium	80 mg
Carbohydrates	47 g	Zinc	2 mg
Protein	23 g	Vitamin E	8 mg
Fiber	9 g		

Strawberry Shake

Here's a smoothie rich in phytoestrogens and vitamin C.

1 cup skim milk

1 cup frozen strawberries

1 banana

2 tablespoons soy protein

1 teaspoon flaxseed oil

1 teaspoon brewer's yeast

Calories	342	Iron	4 mg
Calories from fat	59	Zinc	2 mg
Total fat	7 g	Vitamin B6	1 mg
Carbohydrates	50 g	Folic acid	194 mcg
Protein	25 g	Vitamin C	97 mg
Fiber	6 g		

Banana Shake

This drink makes a good base for herbal supplements.

1 cup vanilla or chocolate soy milk

1 frozen banana, cut into pieces

2 tablespoons vanilla protein powder

1 teaspoon flaxseed powder

Calories	301	Fiber	5 g
Calories from fat	51	Iron	4 mg
Total fat	6 g	Magnesium	46 mg
Carbohydrates	43 g	Potassium	467 mg
Protein	24 g	Vitamin B6	0.7 mg

Green Gardens

Chlorophyll is the green pigment found in plants. It is an excellent source of vitamin K.

1 cup vanilla soy milk

1 tablespoon vanilla soy protein powder

1 tablespoon flaxseed powder

1 teaspoon chlorophyll

1 teaspoon brewer's yeast

Calories	171	Fiber	2 g
Calories from fat	44	Iron	4 mg
Total fat	5 g	Niacin	1 mg
Carbohydrates	17 g	Thiamin	0.4 mg
Protein	15 g	Folic acid	103 mcg

Ginger Cooler

Sip this drink slowly. The ginger is a natural anti-inflammatory agent that helps to relieve menstrual migraine.

1 apple, cored, peeled, and sliced

1/2 cup filtered water

1/2 cup ice

1 lemon, peeled and seeded

1 (2-inch) piece fresh ginger root, peeled and crushed

Calories	150	Fiber	5 g
Calories from fat	11	Magnesium	48 mg
Total fat	1 g	Potassium	574 mg
Carbohydrates	36 g	Niacin	1 mg
Protein	2 g	Vitamin C	40 mg

Tall Red Witch

This unusual tomato-based smoothie is a source of bone-build-ing calcium and phytoestrogens.

1 cup lowfat cottage cheese

1/2 cup tomato juice

1/4 cup tomato paste

1 tablespoon brewer's yeast

1 tablespoon wheat germ

Calories	292	Iron	5 mg
Calories from fat	34	Zinc	2 mg
Total fat	4 g	Folic acid	400 mcg
Carbohydrates	30 g	Beta carotene	2186 mcg
Protein	36 g	Vitamin E	5 mg
Fiber	4 g		

Pumpkin Shake

Pumpkin puree is a wonderful source of beta carotene, which the body turns into vitamin A.

1/2 cup canned pumpkin puree

1/4 cup silken tofu

1 cup vanilla soy milk or skim milk

1 tablespoon blackstrap molasses

1 teaspoon pumpkin pie spice

Calories	245	Calcium	325 mg
Calories from fat	52	Iron	9 mg
Total fat	6 g	Magnesium	72 mg
Carbohydrates	40 g	Vitamin A	2705 mcg
Protein	11 g	Beta carotene	3717 mcg
Fiber	7 g		

Cocoa Berry

Chocolate and strawberries make this smoothie a wonderful way to get your calcium supplements.

1 cup frozen strawberries

1 cup fortified whole soy milk

2 tablespoons chocolate syrup

Calcium/magnesium supplement (see label for
  recommended dosage)

Calories	258	Iron	3 mg
Calories from fat	50	Magnesium	69 mg
Total fat	6 g	Vitamin B12	3 mcg
Carbohydrates	44 g	Vitamin C	85 mg
Protein	12 g	Vitamin E	8 mg
Fiber	8 g		

Berrymint

Mint may help to relieve menstrual cramps. Plant some in a windowsill garden so that there are always fresh leaves available.

1 cup frozen raspberries

1 cup orange juice

4 to 6 mint leaves

Calcium/magnesium supplement (see label for recommended dosage)

Calories	176	Magnesium	49 mg
Calories from fat	8	Potassium	684 mg
Total fat	1 g	Niacin	2 mg
Carbohydrates	42 g	Folic acid	146 mcg
Protein	3 g	Vitamin C	129 mg
Fiber	9 g		

Leaping Lisa

This smoothie is a good source of isoflavones.

1 cup mango slices

1/2 cup silken tofu

1 cup fresh pineapple juice

1 teaspoon flaxseed powder

1 teaspoon flaxseed oil

Calories	404	Iron	5 mg
Calories from fat	106	Vitamin C	73 mg
Total fat	12 g	Vitamin A	656 mcg
Carbohydrates	68 g	Beta carotene	565 mcg
Protein	12 g	Vitamin E	1 mg
Fiber	4 g		

Index

International Conversion Chart

These are not exact equivalents: they have been slightly rounded to make measuring easier.

LIQUID MEASUREMENTS

American	Imperial	Metric	Australian
2 tablespoons (1 oz.)	1 fl. oz.	30 ml	1 tablespoon
1/4 cup (2 oz.)	2 fl. oz.	60 ml	2 tablespoons
1/3 cup (3 oz.)	3 fl. oz.	80 ml	1/4 cup
1/2 cup (4 oz.)	4 fl. oz.	125 ml	1/3 cup
2/3 cup (5 oz.)	5 fl. oz.	165 ml	1/2 cup
3/4 cup (6 oz.)	6 fl. oz.	185 ml	2/3 cup
1 cup (8 oz.)	8 fl. oz.	250 ml	3/4 cup

SPOON MEASUREMENTS

American	Metric
1/4 teaspoon	1 ml
1/2 teaspoon	2 ml
1 teaspoon	5 ml
1 tablespoon	15 ml

WEIGHTS

US/UK	Metric
1 oz.	30 grams (g)
2 oz.	60 g
4 oz. (1/4 lb)	125 g
5 oz. (1/3 lb)	155 g
6 oz.	185 g
7 oz.	220 g
8 oz. (1/2 lb)	250 g
10 oz.	315 g
12 oz. (3/4 lb)	375 g
14 oz.	440 g
16 oz. (1 lb)	500 g
2 lbs	1 kg

OVEN TEMPERATURES

Farenheit	Centigrade	Gas
250	120	1/2
300	150	2
325	160	3
350	180	4
375	190	5
400	200	6
450	230	8

SMOOTHIES FOR EVERYONE!

Low-Carb Smoothies
1-4000-8230-7
$12.95 paper (Canada: $17.95)

Sinful Smoothies
0-7615-2582-3
$12.95 paper (Canada: $19.95)

Slim Smoothies
0-7615-2059-7
$12.95 paper (Canada: $19.95)

Summer Smoothies
0-7615-3732-5
$12.95 paper (Canada: $19.95)

Tipsy Smoothies
0-7615-2650-1
$13.95 paper (Canada: $19.95)